RELIGION AND PAIN

RELIGION
AND PAIN

The Spiritual Dimensions
of Health Care

Joseph H. Fichter

CROSSROAD • NEW YORK

1981
The Crossroad Publishing Company
575 Lexington Avenue, New York, NY 10022

Printed in the United States of America

Library of Congress Cataloging in Publication Data

Fichter, Joseph Henry, 1908–
    Religion and pain.

    Includes index.
    1. Medicine and religion.   2. Pain.   3. Suffering.
4.   Pastoral medicine.   I.   Title.
BL65.M4F52   306'.6   81-7827
ISBN 0-8245-0102-0   AACR2

σταυρῷ καὶ ἰατρῷ

Contents

Preface

This book attempts to steer a middle course between medical researchers who are seeking a solution to the puzzle of physical pain, and theological thinkers who continue to wrestle with the mystery of suffering. Though the researchers represent a clinical, empirical, and scientific approach to the treatment and alleviation of pain, they have not found a solution. The theologians of every generation rethink the paradox of a loving and provident God who allows so much misery and anguish, but they tend to fall back on one or another form of the religious faith of Job. For them, the meaning of pain remains among the insoluble mysteries of religion.

There is not much that a sociologist can do with either the medical or the theological study of human physical pain. Textbooks and courses in medical sociology typically ignore the spiritual dimension of health care, or relegate it to superstitious and magical practices. The usual academic course in social problems devotes considerable attention to the extent of sickness and disease in our society, and to the maldistribution of hospitals and clinics, doctors, nurses, and dentists. Besides teaching such a sociology course annually for many years, I have also conducted a research study of the charismatic movement, in which the power of healing is an important element, and an in-depth field study of the rehabilitation of clergy alcoholics, who also have known great pain. In both of these areas, religion is an important factor in meeting the pervasive problem of human pain and suffering. It is not a difficult transition, then, to move from the study of ill health as a social problem, and from organized movements like Pentecostalism and Alcoholics Anonymous, to the specific sociological analysis of religion-inspired health care.

The practical beginnings of the present research study stem from a conversation with Flavian Dougherty and Cassian Yuhaus, priest members of the Congregation of the Passion and representatives of an international association called *Stauros*. This organization was founded in 1973, the same year that the International Association for the Study of Pain held its Symposium on Pain in Seattle.

The Stauros group directs prayerful and devotional attention to the suffering of Christ and promotes theological study of the gospel of Jesus' passion. At that time, plans were under way for an ecumenical congress of ascetical theologians and biblical scholars to explore the meaning of human suffering in relation to the passion and death of Christ. It was proposed that I do a parallel sociological survey, or opinion poll, to test the hypothesis that American Christians have neglected the "Theology of the Cross," not only in their daily behavior but even in periods of illness, pain, and grief. Whether this ambitious survey of public opinion was viable, and whether its findings would have been useful to the scholars at the congress, adequate funding was not at hand to do the research. Nevertheless, the International Ecumenical Congress on Human Suffering was held at the University of Notre Dame in April, 1979, with almost three hundred participants from sixteen countries and from a diversity of Christian churches.

Seeking a more modest and workable level, I decided to avoid the theological and ascetical area of discussion and to focus on people who are spiritually motivated to deal with the sick on a daily basis. I assumed that if the spiritual dimensions of sick care were to be found anywhere in the country they ought to be discovered in church-related hospitals, those places that were established precisely for the purpose of practicing the corporal and spiritual works of mercy. This, then, is a sociological investigation into cultural patterns and social roles: what do Christian health professionals actually do in the name of religion to comfort the afflicted, to bring the consolations of religion to people on their sick bed?

We are focusing on the health professional, the caretaker, and the healer, not on the person who needs care and seeks healing. Some studies have been made from the perspective of sick patients themselves, investigating how they respond to pain, and whether faith, spirituality, God, religion are in any way a part of that response. In this study, we ask no questions of sick people. We ask rather what kind of religious response do Christian believers make to the sickness and suffering of their fellow human beings. In other words, what is the spiritual dimension of health care, and how does it enter into the remedial treatment of patients? Does modern medical practice take seriously the holistic approach to illness, which includes the spiritual as well as the physical, psychological, and social aspects of the human personality?

Discussions about the relationship between religion and medicine, or between the clergy and the doctors, usually center around ethical problems. What does religion say about informed consent, tubal ligations, and the right to die with dignity? The nurse who refuses to assist at an abortion, the physician who continues (or discontinues) the life-support apparatus of a dying patient are involved in ethical behavior that may be guided by religious convictions. Church-related hospitals have traditionally maintained a strict moral code governing the medical ethics of all affiliated health professionals. Books and articles, conferences and symposia have brought together the representatives of the seminary and the medical school, the hospital and the church, religion and medicine. The Hastings Institute, among others, is paying sophisticated and detailed attention to these ethical problems.

The perspective of this book is the "handling of pain" by people who are spiritually motivated. Our basic assumption is that religion and spirituality are formally integrated with medicine and nursing not only in the large system of church-related hospitals but also in the pastoral-care departments of other voluntary and community hospitals. While gathering the data for this study, I was invited to direct a year-long research project with the Washington-based Center for Applied Research in the Apostolate (CARA). One aspect of the project was to investigate the manner in which four kinds of general voluntary hospitals were achieving the national health priorities set by the United States Congress in Public Law 93–641. This required an on-site visit and extensive interviewing at four health facilities: Mid-Maine Medical Center, Waterville; Greenville Hospital System, Greenville, South Carolina; Presbyterian Hospital Center, Albuquerque, New Mexico; and the Santa Rosa Medical Center, San Antonio, Texas.

The CARA project had a much wider scope than our specific study of religion and pain, but we found much supportive data on the spiritual dimensions of health care in the chaplains' departments maintained at these hospitals. The concept of a therapeutic community is exemplified generally in all American church-related hospitals, but we had to reduce the study to manageable proportions. Because of limited resources, both financial and in personnel, and for the sake of convenience, I decided to focus on a large sample of Catholic general hospitals. Observation and interviews were mainly supplementary to the mass of data obtained through questionnaires.

The preliminary and exploratory stage of this study was a series of visits to hospitals, pain clinics, and doctors' offices. Between March and October, 1978, we taped lengthy interviews with key personnel (nineteen chaplains, fifteen nurses, eleven physicians, and two social workers). With the generous cooperation of two hospital chaplains, Bernard Nugent and Lee Zimmermann, we developed from these discussions a tentative questionnaire. The contents on the survey instrument were pretested and revised on the advice of these professionals before the questionnaire (see Appendix) was mailed. In this way, the pertinent items for the study emerged from the long experience of people who had dedicated their lives and talents to the care of the sick.

From the listings in Kenedy's *Official Catholic Directory,* we selected every other general hospital (excluding sanatoria and special hospitals)—thus sampling exactly half of them—and mailed three questionnaires to the chief executive officer of each. This means that we tried to reach 975 health professionals in 325 hospitals. It required a second or a third mailing to those from whom the responses were slow in coming, but it is a remarkable fact that we have usable answered questionnaires from 92.3 percent of these hospitals. The individual respondents (692) equaled 71 percent of the personnel sample. For the task of processing the research data, we had the invaluable assistance of Daniel Kileen and Zoila Davis at the Computer Center of Tulane University. The computer runs provide a firm foundation for our research report, but we decided to use them in an interpretive mode rather than for precise statistical analysis.

The qualitative interpretation of the questionnaire data was greatly enhanced in two ways. The first was through the interviews, conversations, and observations we were able to make on the CARA hospital research program, which included non-Catholic hospitals. This provided an extraordinary and unanticipated opportunity to dovetail two parallel sociological investigations, each contributing facts and insights to the other. It enabled us to tap analyses and interpretations that represented decades of experience in hospitals, clinics, and hospices. It would be difficult and misleading to name only some—and omit others—of the administrators, chaplains, nurses, physicians, social workers, and psychiatrists who readily contributed their knowledge to this research program. Without their assistance, this report would have resulted in typically disembodied statistics and mathematical formulae.

The second way of bringing the research data alive was by a thorough search of the contemporary literature dealing with the spiritual dimensions of health care. The medical journals and the periodicals in the health profession generally publish very little on this topic. *The Accreditation Manual for Hospitals* (1980 ed.), which is the official publication of the Joint Commission on Accreditation of Hospitals (JCAH) provides no criteria for pastoral-care departments of hospitals. The main source of information is in the publications of the Protestant Hospital Association and the Catholic Health Association. Some reports of careful research studies are available, but many of the articles and pamphlets are on the level of spiritual advice and exhortation.

The review of literature was done faithfully and persistently by my longtime research assistant, Yolanda Hurtado, who combed the libraries for every scrap of information pertinent to this study. At the same time, Michelle Comiskey and Beatrice Michals transcribed into readable typescript the many hours of taped interviews that became an essential ingredient of the research project. The final version of the book was typed with expert care by Patricia Strott. The last word on the enigma of pain has not been said by either the medical researchers or the theological thinkers. This modest investigation reveals, however, that large numbers of religious people dedicate both spiritual compassion and professional competence to the care of suffering patients. Whatever errors, defects, or misinterpretations appear in this research report are the sole responsibility of the author.

Joseph H. Fichter

RELIGION AND PAIN

Chapter 1
Pain: A Source of Religion

There is a popular tendency in much of American religion to play down the sad and somber aspects of human existence. Even the religious liturgies at funerals and burials now have an optimistic note of joyful expectation in eternal life, and some Christians seem to have forgotten that the suffering of their Savior was considered a necessary prelude to the joyful Resurrection. Perhaps the most vocal example of this pattern of cheerful religion is found among the various kinds of Pentecostals. For them, the exciting historical event is the descent of the Holy Spirit forty days after Easter. Born again in the baptism of the Spirit, they turn to glossolalia for the expression of praise and glory to God.

This Pentecostal attitude toward the realities of the human condition is not a denial of pain and suffering; it is a profound conviction that God is at hand to solve all problems and to assume all human burdens. This is the essence of faith healing, which is no longer an exclusive property of lower-class fundamentalists. Charismatics now abound in the mainline Protestant churches as well as among the Episcopalians and Roman Catholics. The central joyful concept is that God can really heal anyone who is suffering, and the key slogan is that "God wants you to be well." [1] Pentecostals emphasize a completely different concept from that which through the ages taught believers to suffer patiently and even to embrace pain as a blessing from God.

The Meaning of Suffering

There is no question that religion has a soothing, calming quality and can be used to maximize joyful celebration and happy thanksgiving, but it has also a more somber side in attempting to handle the tragedies and mysteries of living. The Second Vatican Council made the contrast between joys and hopes on the one hand, and griefs and anxieties on the other. "Though mankind today is struck with wonder at its own discoveries and its power, it often raises anxious questions about the current trend of the world, about the place and role of man in the universe, about the meaning of his individual strivings, and about the ultimate destiny of reality and humanity." [2]

It is probably the "anxious questions" more frequently than the joyful answers that turn people to God and religion. We gladly accept without question the good things in life; but tragedies and anxieties are often incomprehensible. We question them; they are mysteries for which we constantly seek meaning. Clifford Geertz has noted that the problem of suffering is an "experiential challenge in whose face the meaningfulness of a particular pattern of life threatens to dissolve into a chaos of thingless names and nameless things." He suggests further that "as a religious problem, the problem of suffering is, paradoxically, not how to avoid suffering, but how to suffer, how to make of physical pain, personal loss, worldly defeat, or the helpless contemplation of others' agony something bearable, supportable—something, as we say, sufferable." [3]

Anthropologists and psychologists are limited by the very nature of behavioral science to seek functional explanations for the existence of religion. Unlike theologians, who turn to revelation for their basic data, the behavioral scientists may speculate about the origins of religion among the primitives. This indeed is sometimes little more than speculation because prehistoric peoples have left few records and preliterate peoples have handed down only hazy fables from their ancestors. Freud was nevertheless correct, even in modern times, in observing that the terrors, the sufferings, and the hardships of life force some people to turn to religion.[4] Robert Lowie and other anthropologists have hypothesized that religion arose among early human beings when they had to face mysterious, perilous, and terrifying experiences.[5] They searched for meaning above and beyond the phenomena that seemed to have no human or natural explanation.

There is no scientific or causal-historical answer to the question "why must there be suffering in the world?" The specific cause of a specific pain could be sometimes detected, but the larger answer could not be found at the level of natural logic and scientific causality. Behavioral scientists assume then that primitive peoples lifted the question into the realm of supernatural religion. Bypassing the definition of religion and the description of God, the temptation is to paraphrase the "unknown causes" about which David Hume speculated. "We hang in personal suspense between life and death, health and sickness, plenty and want, which are distributed amongst the human species by secret and unknown causes, whose operation is often unexpected, and always unaccountable." [6]

These unknown causes have an intimation of ultimacy about them because they are postulated of the "ultimate conditions" of human existence, and they arise from the "ultimate frustrations of the human situation," as Robert Bellah remarks,[7] and are applied to the "ultimate destiny" of humanity, of which the Second Vatican Council speaks. Life is full of uncertainties. People tend to die at the wrong time; sickness seems to occur when it is most inconvenient; accidents are by definition unexpected. These phenomena entail ultimate problems because they often have no this-worldly explanation. Paul Tillich said that "religion is the state of being grasped by an ultimate concern, a concern which qualifies all other concerns as preliminary and which itself contains the answer to the question of the meaning of life." The otherwise inexplicable and ultimate problems of life lead us to a realization that God is the "predominant religious name for the content of such concern." [8]

The person who does not accept religion on the basis of divine revelation, or the evidence of Scripture, or the message from pulpit preaching may come to some notion of religious reality as the only way to make sense out of pain and suffering. Human experience does not satisfactorily explain the prevalence of human misery. People often turn to religion as they struggle with these problems. J. Milton Yinger writes that religion "expresses their refusal to capitulate to death, to give up in the face of frustration, to allow hostility to tear apart their human associations. The quality of being religious, seen from the individual point of view, implies two things: first, a belief that evil, pain, bewilderment, and injustice are fundamental facts of existence; and, second, a set of practices and related sanctified beliefs that express a conviction that man can ultimately be saved from these facts." [9]

Despite the marvels of technology, and the enormous advance in scientific knowledge, there still remains the nagging mystery of human existence in a world beset with dangers and insecurities. The paradise promised by science has not eventuated; the miseries and anxieties are still there, and seem to be multiplying. Do we have to turn to religion to find whether there is something more than this, whether there is an explanation, whether things could be better? As Yinger asks: "Does life have some central meaning despite the suffering and the succession of frustrations and tragedies it brings?" [10] This is the kind of question that human beings have been asking all through history, perhaps even more so in times and places where life was much more nasty and brutish than most of us experience it in America.

At this level of reflection there is no attempt to reproduce Thomas Aquinas's five proofs for the existence of God, or Saint Anselm's ontological argument. Part of the mystery of suffering is the odd maldistribution of pain, with some people undergoing almost intolerable misery, while others seem to live in the midst of good health and good fortune. Some people are intellectually more perceptive than others and may be capable of greater insights into the human condition. No one needs a leap of faith to recognize the existence of pain and misery. The willingness, however, to admit that there *has* to be some meaning to human suffering is merely the first step in acknowledging that the meaning is beyond human comprehension. It is then a mystery, and mysteries belong in the realm of religion.

Pain and Religious Belief

The purpose of this study is not to explain the varieties of pain or to trace the origins of religion in the attempt to understand the significance of suffering. Nevertheless, the theoretical functional explanation why religion continues to exist in the highly secularized contemporary society is that it provides some meaning to the otherwise meaningless experience of human suffering. While pain is unquestionably felt by brute animals, the puzzle of its meaning is a question for human beings. Victor Frankl observed that a laboratory ape being "punctured again and again would never be able to grasp the meaning of its suffering." Then he asked the transcendent question about people. "Are you sure that the human world is a terminal point in the evolution of the cosmos? Is it not conceivable that there is still another dimension possible, a world beyond man's world; a world in which the question of an ultimate meaning of human suffering would find an answer?" [11] The obvious direction of this trend of questioning is that the ultimate answer has to be found in the future life of which the preachers speak and the Scripture scholars write, and to which religious believers aspire.

The religious believer foresees a future life in which the mysteries will be clarified. People are constantly trying to understand what life is all about, and why so much occurs that is unexpected and unaccountable and undesirable. Not everyone develops religious beliefs out of this puzzling situation, nor is there necessarily a close similarity in the religious concepts that do evolve from such experience. Nevertheless, as Talcott Parsons observed, "religion has its greatest relevance to the points of maximum strain and tension in human life as well as to positive affirmations of faith in life, often in the face of these strains." [12]

The reasons *why* people profess a religious belief of some kind do not necessarily define the content or the general mode of their belief. In some past centuries when large numbers of the population experienced plague and famine, their religious response was characterized by penitential practices, doleful liturgies, concern about sin and punishment. The death rate was high; life was short, cruel, and hard, and the prospect of a religion of eternal salvation kept people from despair. Believers prayed for divine mercy and forgiveness of their sins and deliverance from the bonds of sin and Satan. Their preachers talked about this temporal "vale of tears," about the trials and tribulations and temptations that had to be overcome. Religion then meant to them a redemption from sin as well as from suffering.

Contemporary existence, at least for large numbers of people in western society, tends to embody a less pessimistic interpretation of life's misfortunes. The miseries and anxieties are just as prevalent and may be even more baffling because there is a greater expectation that human effort can do more to alleviate suffering and pain. But the mystery remains and it logically seeks an answer in religion, even though the content of the religion tends to be more cheerful. This fact of cultural influence is not to suggest that a sad religion is more likely—or less likely—to be "true" than a joyful religion. It must be noted also that the social scientist, relying only on his empirical, testable data, does not presume to judge the truth of any religion.

In other words, this "naturalistic" manner of coming to religion through the experience of pain and suffering is not the only reason why people acknowledge some supernatural power, nor is it necessarily the only doorway to religion. On the other hand, this experiential approach seems still to be the path along which large numbers of modern puzzled people search for meaning. People who adhere to the revealed religion of the Judeo-Christian tradition may tend to downgrade these "primitive" concepts. It should be noted that the Second Vatican Council called attention to the fact that people in non-Christian religions

everywhere "strive variously to answer the restless search-
ings of the human heart." [13] Thus the natural human search
for answers to the mystery of existence is not to be faulted
or spurned. This "restless searching" for answers to life's
puzzles is seen as a universal experience regardless of religious traditions. It cannot be suggested, therefore, that the
Council was belittling divine inspiration, revelation, and
tradition when it declared that people "look to the various
religions for answers to those profound mysteries of the
human condition which, today even as in olden times,
deeply stir the human heart: what is man? What is the
meaning and purpose of our life? What is goodness and
what is sin? What gives rise to our sorrow and to what intent? Where lies the path to true happiness? What is the
truth about death, judgment, and retribution beyond the
grave?" [14]

The profound mysteries of life are discussed and
explored by persons other than ministers and priests, and
often enough by psychological counselors. Victor Frankl
noted that the religious question of meaning is often asked
of the physician rather than of the clergyman. "What is life?
What is suffering after all? Indeed, incessantly and con-
tinually a psychiatrist is approached today by patients who
confront him with human problems rather than neurotic
symptoms. Some of the people who nowadays call on a
psychiatrist would have seen a pastor, priest, or rabbi in
former days, but now they often refuse to be handed over to
a clergyman, so that the doctor is confronted with
philosophical questions rather than emotional conflicts." [15]

Finding a philosophical answer to a philosophical question is not the same as making a religious response to the
actual experience of pain. The earliest physician of record,
Hippocrates, is said to have philosophized about the causes
of sickness and the nature of healing, and concluded that
epilepsy is of divine origin. In more recent times, some
sociologists have unhesitatingly embraced supraempirical
postulates like the existence of God and the immortality of
the human soul.[16] Even Karl Marx recognized the function

of religion in the lives of the suffering people. He was not merely engaged in abstract speculations when he observed economically deprived peasants staggering under the burdens of social injustice. He was willing to say that "religion is the sigh of the oppressed creature, the heart of a heartless world, the soul of soulless conditions." [17]

Inexplicable Suffering

Religious people, too, are deeply concerned about exploitation and social injustice. The social gospel movement among Protestants at the turn of the century, the concurrent publication of papal social encyclicals, and the frequent insistence that the search for social justice is a constitutive element of evangelization provide evidence that the sources of exploitation can be recognized and attacked. In other words, the pain that is visited on people by racists, by unjust employers, by selfish exploiters, is not a matter of inexplicable mystery. Throughout history, some people have been oppressed by others, in slavery, in bondage, and in poverty. It may be impossible to obtain redress in many instances, but it is often possible to point the finger of accusation at the perpetrator of pain.

Police statistics indicate a steady increase in urban crimes against the person, unprovoked acts of violence, apparently random attacks on ordinary citizens. Here again, the cause of pain can be traced to the person who accidentally or deliberately hurts another. The "mystery" may lie in the motivation of the attackers, whether or not under the influence of drugs, and if this cannot be discovered we commonly talk of "senseless" cruelty. There are, of course, countless intentional acts of criminality. The fact that an offender is arrested, brought before the court, found guilty, and sentenced to some form of legal punishment—this whole process may end with no explanation why the culprit behaved in such fashion.

Even the ravages of destructive warfare, with the senseless bombing of civilians, are not the mysterious source of suffering and pain. Large-scale modern warfare is most often sinful, murderous, and unjust, but its destructiveness can be traced to its source. Wars are managed by human beings. Decisions for killing and destruction are made deliberately. The attendant misery in homeless and displaced population, in hunger, sickness, and death, may be termed unfortunate "side effects" of warfare. Believers may ask why a just and loving God "allows" such heinous crimes, even while they know that human beings committed the crimes.

What can one say about "natural" catastrophes that were not caused by human beings? Volcanos, earthquakes, typhoons, and other kinds of storms may have been mysterious to primitives, who were inspired to seek their cause in some supernatural force. The anxieties and uncertainties that accompanied such misfortunes made them turn to a higher power in their lives. Modern science cannot predict with any degree of accuracy the occurrence of such natural catastrophes, but the physical forces unleashed in them are fairly well understood. Even a drought or a flood is "blamed" for the dire suffering it brings to people, but these are no longer considered "mysterious" or inexplicable causes of calamity.

It should be noted, however, that human beings sometimes bring suffering on themselves. The person who wakes up with a "hangover" may not remember clearly the happenings of the previous evening but does recognize the source of the headache. The constant and overuse of drugs to kill pain may itself lead to painful addiction. Alcoholism is a sickness that can be traced directly to overindulgence and often requires almost heroic efforts at rehabilitation. But the cause is known. Some physicians warn that excessive smoking of cigarettes may cause emphysema, and the patient who has this illness need look no further for an explanation. There are probably many other examples of self-inflicted pain that results from culpable, foolish, or thoughtless behavior.

Here we are talking about personal bodily pain, which is "localizable" as a sensation but is not objectively measurable by observer, nurse, or clinician.[18] Most of the patients who are treated at the hospitals covered by this study are under treatment because they suffer some recognizable injury, sickness, or disease. When we ask about sick care and about the spiritual dimensions of medical service we are specifically looking at the kind of pain that is an unexplained mystery. It is a puzzle that involves three characteristics: such pain is perceived by the individual patient as personal, unexpected, and undeserved.

Since pain is an experience that touches and envelops the whole person it is not easily distinguished into bodily pain and mental pain, although this distinction is frequently made in ordinary conversation.[19] For the purpose of this study, we focus mainly on pain that is immediate and physical and cannot be shared with any other individual, no matter how compassionate or loving that person may be. In dealing with sick people, we want to avoid theoretical explanations—which would be about as useful for the sufferer as a lecture on cholesterol is for a starving person.

This level of personal pain becomes mysterious and inexplicable precisely to the extent that it is also unexpected and undeserved. The patient who anticipates pain on the morning before a surgical operation has usually been informed why an operation is necessary, what it is intended to accomplish, and also that this is an intervention in the normal functioning of the human body. Nothing is totally mysterious if it is anticipated. Nevertheless, the questioning patient is found in every hospital. More frequently than any other health professional, it is the nurse who hears the cry: "Why is this happening to me? Why do I have to suffer like this?"

Pain is more puzzling to the extent that it is undeserved. The most dramatic examples are known to all of us: the child born with some handicap or deformity, the adult with an incurable disease not traceable to any cause, the person severely injured in an accident for which no one is at fault. The human mind is in quest of meaning, and it is at this point that some religious people feel that God is punishing them. The tendency is to feel guilty—even when there is no guilt. As Geertz remarks, "the problem of suffering easily passes into the problem of evil, for if suffering is severe enough it usually, though not always, seems morally undeserved as well, at least to the sufferer." [20]

Notes

1 Title of the book by Laurence Blackburn, *God Wants You to Be Well* (New York: Morehouse-Barlow, 1970); similarly, Emily Gardiner Neal, *God Can Heal You Now* (Englewood Cliffs: Prentice-Hall, 1958), and Francis MacNutt, *Healing* (Notre Dame: Ave Maria Press, 1974).

2 "The Church in the Modern World," *Gaudium et Spes*, ART. 3.

3 Clifford Geertz, "Religion as a Cultural System," in *Anthropological Approaches to the Study of Religion* ed. Michael Benton (London: Tavistock, 1966), pp. 1–46.

4 Thus in Sigmund Freud, *The Future of An Illusion* (London: Hogarth Press, 1928)

5 Robert Lowie, *Primitive Religion* (New York: Boni and Liveright, 1924).

6 David Hume, "Origin of Religion," in *Sociology and Religion*, ed. Norman Birnbaum and Gertrud Lenzer (Englewood Cliffs: Prentice-Hall, 1969), pp. 19–22.

7 Robert Bellah, *Beyond Belief* (New York: Harper & Row, 1970), p. 275.

8 Paul Tillich, *Christianity and the Encounter of the World Religions* (New York: Columbia University Press, 1963), pp. 4–5.

9 J. Milton Yinger, *The Scientific Study of Religion* (New York: Macmillan, 1970), p. 7.

10 Yinger, *Scientific Study*, p. 6.

11 Victor Frankl, *Man's Search for Meaning* (New York: Simon & Schuster, 1972), p. 187.

12 Talcott Parsons, "Sociology and Social Psychology," in *Religious Perspectives in College Teaching*, ed. Hoxie Fairchild (New York: Ronald Press, 1952), pp. 293–99.

13 "On Non-Christian Religions," *Nostra Aetate*, ART. 2

14 Ibid., ART. 1

15 Frankl, *Man's Search*, pp. 183–84. Another physician admits to a "mismatch" between his professional preparation and the kinds of questions asked by people in need, "basic religious questions, such as, What is human life for?" Donald W. Shriver, "The Interrelationships of Religion and Medicine," in *Medicine and Religion*, ed. Donald W. Shriver (Pittsburgh: University of Pittsburgh Press, 1980), pp. 21–45.

16 A "metasociological treatise" was developed by Paul Hanly Furfey, *The Scope and Method of Sociology* (New York: Harper and Brothers, 1953). His theory of value judgments has been revived by some younger sociologists in recent years.

17 Karl Marx, "Contribution to the Critique of Hegel's Philosophy of Right," in Karl Marx and Friedrich Engels, *On Religion* (London: Lawrence and Wishart, 1957), pp. 41–42.

18 This is a common definition discussed by E. L. Edelstein, "Experience and Mastery of Pain," *Israel Annals of Psychiatry and Related Disciplines* (September 1974): 216–26.

19 The varying vocabulary for the concepts of pain and suffering in different languages is footnoted in Mark Zborowski, *People in Pain* (San Francisco: Jossey-Bass, 1969), pp. 38–39.

20 Geertz, "Religion as a Cultural System," p. 21.

Chapter 2
Secular Response to Pain

If religion strives to understand the meaning of pain and the reasons why suffering continues to be a widespread human experience, medical science strives to get rid of pain, or to alleviate it as far as possible. Theology and science have learned to live together, and it is said that religion and medicine must complement each other.[1] There is a tendency, however, to overestimate the medical profession as all-wise and all-powerful in the face of suffering. "In our era of deification of technological science," writes Edelstein, "pain is considered by people as a superfluous nuisance." [2] Whether or not the consolations of religion are able to relieve suffering, the fact is that medical science has made great strides in reducing the intensity of physical pain.

Still, the maldistribution of health professionals and of clinics and hospitals, even in advanced western countries, leaves large numbers of sick people with only rare recourse to health-care facilities, and for them pain is something more than a "superfluous nuisance." Public frustration is expressed over these inadequacies in a nation that prides itself on its enormous organizational and technical talent.[3] Another kind of frustration exists at the level of recognition of limitations in medical research and therapy. Even in a first-rate research hospital it could be said that "since the knowledge and skills of the physician are not always adequate, there are many times when his most vigorous efforts to understand illness and to rectify its consequences are of little or no avail." [4]

Alleviating Pain

Pain is real to the person who feels it, and there is no way that another person can truly measure it or genuinely share it. Pain is always a personal experience that differs in intensity from individual to individual, but it can be recognized, analyzed, and discussed in several categories. The most common preliminary distinction is to define suffering separately from pain. One may "suffer" many losses—of friends, of money, of reputation—and at the same time may not be in any bodily discomfort. Suffering may be described also as the emotional, subjective, and evaluative response that most often accompanies physical pain. It has been observed by experienced clinicians that when suffering is allayed, or removed, "pure pain" does not hurt so much.[5]

It will be difficult to keep these two concepts separate in this book because we frequently heard nurses and doctors talk about the "imaginary" pain of patients, the most spectacular being that of the amputated limb, the extremity of which still hurts. There are, however, many other cases in which pain is felt, or amplified, through apprehension, fear, anxiety, or worry. Many people suffer pain that does not seem to have an organic source. The skilled nurse recognizes the need for allaying this kind of "pain," and it is not done with medication. "This is something you learn through experience, and not in the nursing school." Many nurses have told us that the nonmedical aspects of nursing take more time and skill than the strictly technical aspects. Modern researchers are paying close attention to the kinds of pain that seem to have a nonorganic basis. One research psychologist comments: "I'm interested in how people make themselves sick and how they make themselves well, and I'm beginning to think that a great deal of what medicine contends with is exactly that. Of course, one can't explain all problems in this way, but I suspect that a substantial portion of patients fall into this category. People seek help because they are sick, and in some cases they've either made themselves sick foolishly, or they've done it intentionally at some subconscious level. A great deal of what we call cure, even if it follows neurosurgical intervention, occurs because the patient is now ready to change his life and get rid of what he was doing before." [6]

Similar comments were made frequently by physicians we interviewed. One busy and experienced internist told us: "A lot of patients are not at peace with themselves. They claim they are hurting but there is not much wrong with them. Like the lady who has a chest cold and insists that it is pneumonia and she has to go to the hospital. I would say that half the people who are in the hospital are there because of reasons other than pure physical illness. I keep saying they are not at peace with themselves; they are depressed and disturbed, and have all kinds of other problems that can't be cured with pain shots." For the most part we think of hospitals and sick beds as places that people ordinarily want to avoid, but we have testimony about patients who could have had day surgery but insisited on admission to the hospital and later "enjoyed" telling their friends about the experience.

There is another distinction that sometimes arises in discussions about the healing of people in pain. This is the question of the difference between care and cure of hospital patients. We are told that "ideally, the nurse should have charge over the care for the patient." [7] One physician insists there should be more emphasis on care than on cure: "The primary and ultimate functions of a physician are the alleviation of human suffering. All-consuming obsession with cure of the sick more often that not leads to recurrent frustrations in the doctor so limited in his perspectives, and to disappointment and disillusion in his ill-informed patients." [8] All of the hospital personnel we interviewed said they try to be optimistic in the care of their patients but are careful not to promise their complete cure. Out of their experience grows a cautious understanding that when a cure does occur it may sometimes be the result of factors beyond the intervention of the medical staff and even beyond scientific explanation. Often enough the best the physician can do is to assuage the distress of the patient, to lessen the intensity of the pain. Always, however, it is the function of all sick-care professionals to bring comfort to the suffering. The practical aspirations of the medical profession are expressed then in the "old axiom" quoted by Zuromskis: *guérir parfois, soulager souvent, consoler toujours.*

Americans particularly have come to expect the alleviation of pain, and even to demand instant relief of the minor aches and ailments that accompany everyday living. It is a reflection of contemporary culture that we are impatient with any degree of discomfort. TV commercials constantly assault us with the magic of pills of all kinds to relieve pain, lessen nervousness, guarantee sleep. There is no need to pay the price for self-indulgence that results in indigestion or hangovers. The warning "to take only as directed" is, of course, always included, as is the suggestion to see a physician if it does not work. What this means is that drugs are readily available, and over-the-counter medications are sold in every corner store and every supermarket. Commercial pharmaceutical companies have poured out an endless stream of nostrums and anodynes for practically any kind of discomfort human beings experience. Some of the advertising is questionable and some of the claims are exaggerated, but immediate and even "long-lasting" relief is promised for headaches, arthritis, catarrh, neuralgia, and a multitude of other identifiable aches in the everyday life of people. Thus the phenomenal success—not to speak of the extraordinary financial profit—that has accompanied the production and distribution of pain suppressants and the glowing promises invented by admen tend to make sick people impatient for a quick cure when they experience genuine, serious, and intractable pain.

Levels of Pain

The experience of pain ranges from the temporary to the terminal, from the imaginary to the genuine, from the trivial to the serious, and the attitude toward suffering shifts from generation to generation. Behavioral scientists suggest that we are different from our forebears. The publicity that surrounds medical and surgical "breakthroughs" has raised our health expectations and increased our demands for more attentive doctors, better health facilities, and more hospital services. One expert observer interprets this as a burdensome exaggeration and says "it is as though our health-care consumers have almost a fairy-tale mentality, which refuses to acknowledge the limitations of medicine and the inevitability of some suffering." [9]

Whether one blames the general public for having unreal health expectations or the medical profession, and especially the apothecaries, for making unreal health promises, the fact is that pain is an unpleasant experience at any level, and the great majority of people want to get rid of it as quickly as possible. Medical practitioners generally admit, at least in private conversations, that there is too much and too frequent use of Valium and Librium and other potentially addictive substances, but they may often continue to prescribe such drugs. They say that the ambulatory patient, whether at the doctor's office or the hospital emergency room, demands this kind of attention even when there is no clear diagnosis of a definite ailment. One physician told us that "whether or not they need the medicine, the big advantage is that they do feel better if you give them a prescription." This level of medical care may make the patient "feel good," but it is also very distressing to the conscientious physician and enormously profitable for the manufacturer and distributor of drugs.

The temporary inconvenience and superficial discomfort of those who seek instant relief through pills and drugs are far removed from patients who are terminally ill. This is a different level of suffering, and medical doctors tend to have widely varying attitudes toward patients who cannot be restored to health. The dying patient represents "failure" to medical science, a sign that therapeutic skills were inadequate. Once the physician has "given up" on the dying person, the temptation for even the compassionate medical doctor is to walk away and let the nurse give comfort and attempt to alleviate the final suffering. At this point, even the most areligious physician may call in the hospital chaplain.[10]

The ability to cope with the fact of approaching death, and with the accompanying physical pain, has been explored in several controversial studies by Elisabeth Kubler-Ross.[11] The "stages" through which the dying person moves have been discussed and argued at great length by many people, and there is no doubt that the process is flexible and individualized. Nevertheless, many healthcare professionals share the common view of one nurse who remarked: "Given the amount of pain, and the amount of loss, separation, and distress, their ability to cope with it has been absolutely edifying. I've never been so impressed as I have been with people in those circumstances." Thus, Raymond Carey rightly suggests that hospital personnel who may not be able to relieve the pain should be concerned with helping patients "live each day as joyfully and peacefully as possible." [12]

It is true that in some of the lingering illnesses that lead to death there is relatively little pain, while in other instances the suffering becomes intense. Between these two poles, however, the great majority of dying patients find their suffering alleviated by gradually increased medication. The religious themes of this book do not include items of medical ethics, but it may be noted that the question whether to continue treatment and experimentation, or to allow death to occur, has been the subject of much discussion and even of legislation that assures "death with dignity." [13] Nurses who care for the terminally ill often remark that death ordinarily comes with great apparent peacefulness only because the patients have been heavily and effectively sedated.

Between the category of people who have passing pains or imaginary aches, and those who are enduring their final illness, is the large number of sick people—most of them hospitalized—who will recover from their physical distress and will resume the tasks of normal living. These are the temporary occupants of hospital beds with whom the health-care informants for this study were mostly involved. These are the people hospitalized by their physicians for serious illness, or brought into the emergency room as victims of accidents, or recovering from major surgery. Here again, medical personnel recognize that pain is individual and subjective, and that in some cases it is much more intense than in others.

Everyone who is scheduled for surgery in a hospital is aware that "this is going to hurt." Some degree of pain is inevitably associated with the surgical operation, but tremendous advances have been made in reducing the intensity of the pain. "Relatively speaking," said one compassionate surgeon, "the aftereffects of most surgery are now almost painless. In the old days, the drugs were just not available, but now we are able to alleviate about ninety percent of the pain. But you can't, and you really don't want to, remove pain altogether." The expectation is that ultimately the operation will heal, or the serious sickness will abate, and the pain will disappear. With some patients, however, this expectation is not met and the promise is not kept.

Chronic Pain

The most puzzling sort of pain is that which persists and for which medical science has found neither an explanation nor a permanent cure. The necessary surgery has been performed, all proper medication prescribed, but the medical expert is baffled by the complexity of suffering which goes beyond recognizable bodily symptoms and accessible remedies. Despite all medical efforts to provide relief, the physical suffering continues. Samuel Mines points out that "chronic pain does not become more tolerable with time. On the contrary, pain appears to sensitize the system so that suffering becomes worse the longer it continues." [14] The knotty problem of perennial pain is acknowledged also by Ronald Melzack, who wrote: "It is a fundamental fact in the field of pain that some patients will suffer pain for the rest of their lives. In such cases, the most effective therapy may be to teach them to live with their pain, to carry on productive lives in spite of it." [15] Health-care professionals make a distinction between people who are dying of a known disease like cancer, which is the source of their chronic pain, and people who constantly complain of pain, the source of which cannot be determined. They recognize also the difference between acute pain and chronic pain. John Bonica writes that "whereas acute symptomatic pain serves the useful diagnostic aid for physicians, in its chronic pathologic form, pain is a malefic force which often imposes severe emotional, physical, and economic stress on the patient, on his family, and on society." [16]

Some chronic-pain patients are a source of frustration to medical doctors who examine them carefully and repeatedly and cannot discern objectively why they are undergoing such disproportionate pain. One physician told us with some irritation: "There is a subgroup of these people who have been not only to your pain clinic but also to other pain clinics. They may have had surgery several times. Their interpersonal relations are often distorted and their difficulties are based on psychological sickness; they need to be checked out by a psychiatrist." Some physicians who recognize such people tend to call them "crocks." On the other hand, disgruntled patients who cannot find relief sometimes complain about their doctors as "quacks." Melzack clearly states: "The patient who visits a clinic and is told that he must learn to live with his pain usually concludes that the physician is incompetent and therefore visits doctor after doctor in search for the all-encompassing, perfect pain-control method. The patients with the sick dossiers ('crocks') may, possibly, have deep-seated psychological problems; but they are also a product of our Western all-or-nothing pill-popping ethos, which promises instant, total pain relief—if not now, then to-morrow." [17]

Aside from such people whose pain may be more psychological than physical, the persistent phenomenon of chronic pain has found response in the specialized pain clinics that are being established at more and more hospitals throughout the country. These clinics aim at what C. Norman Shealy calls the "holistic treatment and rehabilitation of patients with chronic intractable pain." The total approach to therapy and pain relief involves an interdisciplinary team which generally includes a neurosurgeon, psychiatrist, physical therapist, neuro-technician, dietician, social worker, and several nurses.[18] A trained chaplain, or spiritual counselor, was a regular member of the team in these pain clinics, with one exception: a church-related hospital which had as its director a neurosurgeon who declared that the chronic-pain patient must be shed of all dependencies. According to his interpretation, religion is a redundant crutch.[19]

There is still another category of sufferers who have real difficulty in reconciling themselves to their painful condition. These are the handicapped, or permanently crippled persons, who became disabled after having once had the full use of their limbs. Much praise and publicity has been given to those exceptional people who continue to have strong religious faith in spite of their disabilities. But it appears that the majority react differently. The chaplain at a large public urban rehabilitation hospital told us: "I see a lot of people turning bitter and losing their faith. That's very common with the handicapped people; they just totally give up on God and religion and faith of any kind. Many of our former patients now say that they are agnostics, or that they are atheists."

The Secular Approach

Pastoral care is provided for the patients in many so-called secular hospitals, whether under private, public, or governmental auspices. The extent to which the spiritual ministry to the sick is accepted as an integral element of the holistic scheme of health care seems to depend largely on the local administration and board of directors of each hospital. The "bible" for these secular hospitals is the *Accreditation Manual*, which "has become the canon by which hospitals have been guided in their pursuit of excellence" and is also the set of standards against which the periodic visiting teams from the Joint Commission on Accreditation of Hospitals measure the local institution.[20] Nowhere in this *Manual* (1980 ed.) is there any mention of pastoral care, or of the spiritual dimension of the healing process. Church-related hospitals seek accreditation from this joint commission, but they also follow the additional criteria written into the constitutions of the Protestant Hospital Association and of the Catholic Health Association.

Nevertheless, quite aside from considerations of religion and spirituality there has been a notable and growing concentration in the world of neurology, medical science, and health care on the problem of physical pain. The International Symposium on Pain, held in Seattle in 1973, was attended by more than 350 physicians, scientists, anesthesiologists, psychotherapists and other health professionals from thirteen countries, who listened to eighty-nine scholarly papers prepared for the occasion. The role of religion was nowhere on the agenda. These scientists presented a clinical and empirical approach to the treatment and alleviation of physical suffering. "There are few problems that are more worthy of human endeavor than the puzzle of pain," wrote Ronald Melzack in his foreword to the symposium proceedings. "Its solution is compelled by the human desire to release pain and suffering, for those who will recover and go on to live useful lives, and for those whose lives are coming to an end." [21] They were not seeking the metaphysical or religious meaning of pain, and they also came away from their meeting without a scientific solution to the puzzle.[22]

The person who is afflicted with chronic pain turns to the pain clinic as a last resort, finds there no quick and magic relief, but is taught how to "manage" pain. Victor Christopherson points out that "the underlying assumption in this approach is that, if pain response is to some extent at least learned behavior, it follows that the individual can also learn to respond in certain predetermined ways to pain as a result of a training or learning process." [23] There is even a gradual withdrawal from medication in the application of this so-called operant-conditioning technique.[24] In essence, however, this is not a medical approach to pain relief, and the person who runs the clinic and teaches this method need not be a trained physician.

People who are admitted to pain clinics tend to be depressed and discouraged, but they are not the pathological "crocks" easily recognized by health-care professionals and screened out of the program. They have a medical history and can usually trace the beginning of their pain to some accidental injury, after which they continued to be under stress and tension. Their treatment is largely a program of behavior modification, but it is not meant merely to teach them how to live with their pain. There is an actual reduction in physical pain through physical therapy and exercise and in the learning process of relaxation. One Sister in charge of a pain clinic said, "it is not just mind over matter. Muscles are relaxing and that lessens the aggravation of pain. That's what biofeedback is all about; they learn to lower that muscle contraction."

It is, of course, too much to expect that all chronic-pain patients can be completely rehabilitated, or that bodily pain can ultimately be entirely avoided, prevented, or removed from humanity. Nevertheless, there are still some people with the "fairy-tale mentality" who continue to make demands for the alleviation of every ache and pain. Scientific research continues by dedicated experts who work ambivalently toward a breakthrough, though many scientists, such as Raymond Fink, are not so sure that a painless existence is completely desirable. "At a time when self-gratification by electrical stimulation of the brain is an accomplished fact, a daily existence rendered universally pain free by artificial means seems a promise (or menace) realizable in the not-so-distant future." [25]

Notes

1 See Bernard Martin, *The Healing Ministry in the Church* (Richmond, Va.: John Knox Press, 1961).

2 E. L. Edelstein, "Experience and Mastery of Pain," *Israel Annals of Psychiatry and Related Disciplines* (September 1974): 216–26.

3 See two articles in the *National Catholic Reporter* for 9 May 1980: Fred McCunagle, "Crusaders Fight For Health of Inner-City Poor," and Mark Neilsen, "Health Care."

4 Renée C. Fox, *Experiment Perilous* (Glencoe: Free Press, 1959), p. 238.

5 David Cheek and Leslie LeCron, "Pain: Its Meaning and Treatment," in *Clinical Hypnotherapy* (New York: Grune & Stratton, 1968), pp. 142–52.

6 C. Richard Chapman, as quoted by Samuel Mines, *The Conquest of Pain* (New York: Grosset & Dunlap, 1974), p. 29. A similar approach is supported in Arnold Hutschnecker, *The Will to Live* (New York: Cornerstone Library, 1974), chap. 8, "We Select Our Illnesses," pp. 95–105.

7 Gerald Niklas and Charlotte Stefanics, *Ministry to the Hospitalized* (New York: Paulist Press, 1975), p. 4.

8 Letter of physician Peter Zuromskis to the editor of *Harvard Magazine* (September–October 1978): 11. The chief of pastoral care at Albuquerque's Presbyterian Hospital writes his book "for those who have to care for the sick." See Dennis Saylor, *And You Visited Me* (Medford: Morse Press, 1979).

9 Serena Branson, "Social Trends Challenge Hospitals," *Hospital Progress* (August 1977): 68–71.

10 Hippocrates taught that the doctor is called by God to relieve pain. "His office is not to console, but to heal." The doctor at the bedside becomes aware that pain is not merely a problem, but a mystery. See the excellent study by F. J. J. Buytendijk, *Pain: Its Modes and Functions* (Chicago: University of Chicago Press, 1962), pp. 40–41.

11 Elisabeth Kubler-Ross, *On Death and Dying* (New York: Macmillan, 1969). Relatives and friends of the dying person are said also to go through "stages in grief." See Myron C. Madden, *Raise the Dead!* (Waco: Word Books, 1975), pp. 36–42. See also the critical theological appraisal by George Kuykendall, "On Caring for the Dying," *Theology Today* (April 1981), pp. 37–48.

12 Raymond Carey, "Counselling the Terminally Ill," *Personnel and Guidance Journal* (November 1976): 124–26.

13 The first American legislation of this kind was the Natural Death Act, signed into law in California in September, 1976. See Thomas Horkan, "Death with Dignity, California Style," *Hospital Progress* 58 (February 1977): 12–13. The moral and legal aspects were later discussed by Nicholas Spinells, "Update on Opposition to Death-with-Dignity Legislation," *Hospital Progress* 58 (July 1977): 70–72, 81.

14 Samuel Mines, *The Conquest of Pain* (New York: Grosset and Dunlap, 1974) p. 9.

15 Ronald Melzack, "Psychological Concepts and Methods for the Control of Pain," in *International Symposium of Pain*, ed. John J. Bonica (New York: Raven Press, 1974), pp. 275–80.

16 Bonica, *International Symposium*, Preface, p. vii. Buytendijk, *Pain*, p. 172, quotes Leriche: "Pain is always a sinister gift. It lowers man and makes him more ill than he would be without it."

17 Ronald Melzack, "Psychological Concepts," p. 277. See also Mines, *Conquest of Pain*, chap. 11, "Pain Games and Alternatives." Thomas Szasz writes cynically about people who "make a career of suffering." See his paper, "The Psychology of Persistent Pain: A Portrait of L'Homme Douloureux," in *Pain*, ed. A. Soulairac, J. Cahn, and J. Charpentier (New York: Academic Press, 1968), pp. 93–113.

18 C. Norman Shealy, *The Pain Game* (Milbrae: Celestial Arts, 1976), also his article, "The Pain Patient," *American Family Physician* (1974): 130–36. It should be noted that Shealy's Pain Health Rehabilitation Center in Wisconsin includes two pastoral counselors on the staff.

19 This director said also that clergymen are not properly trained to work with chronic-pain patients.

20 Representatives of church-related hopsitals are said to have been influential in establishing the joint commission which grew out of this effort in Robert J. Shanahan, *The History of the Catholic Hospital Association* (St. Louis: Catholic Hospital Association, 1965), chap. 2, "Hospital Standardization."

21 Ronald Melzack in Bonica, *International Symposium*, Foreword, p. v.

22 Besides the Seattle symposium in 1973, the National Institute of General Medical Sciences sponsored a world congress on pain in Florence, Italy, in 1975 and another in Montreal in 1978.

There has come into existence also an International Association for the Study of Pain, which has among its members increasing numbers of scientific specialists of all types: anatomists, anesthesiologists, internists, neurologists, neuropharmacologists, physiologists, orthopedists, psychiatrists, psychologists, and surgeons. This organization publishes a journal with the appropriate title, *Pain*.

23 Victor A. Christopherson, "Sociocultural Correlates on Pain Response," *Social Science* (January 1971): 33–37.

24 On drugs and operant conditioning, see Shealy, *Pain Game*, pp. 53–57.

25 B. Raymond Fink, "Pain in Perspective, 1975," *Perspective in Biology and Medicine* 19, no. 2 (Winter 1976): 278–84.

Chapter 3
The Theodicy of Pain

Although medical technology has made great advances in controlling the painful manifestations of injuries and disease, the medical profession has not come to an adequate explanation of the puzzle of pain. Theologians have pondered longer and deepr than physicians, but they continue also to look for the key to the mystery of pain. If the experience of anguish and uncertainty, of pain and misery, has driven humanity to the acceptance of religion, what explanation can religion offer? At some point in their lives, all people "must come to terms with dimensions of human experience that can be confronted only in a religious context." It seems inevitable then, adds Francis Cleary, that "all religious systems must somehow come to grips with this question, and their sacred writings reflect their groping." [1]

Since Leibniz the mystery of suffering has been related to the mystery of God and the combination has been treated as the question of theodicy. In other words, the religious believer has to find a way to defend God's goodness and omnipotence in the face of universal suffering and inexplicable pain. "Life's ultimate questions—and among them are certainly sickness, suffering, and death—must be answered in the light of the fundamental insights of our faith: otherwise the answers are not merely too superficial, but simply false." [2] Contemporary health professionals, by the very nature of their constant contact with suffering people, are logically driven to satisfy this quest. Without attempting to review the endless speculations of spiritual writers on this difficult subject, we may note that the religious response to pain falls into three categories: first, this is a mystery which has no explanation. Second, we may accept pain as a blessing from God. Third, we may reject pain as unintended by God.

The Insoluble Problem

The explanation that comes from theodicy is not a search for causality, but a search for meaning. Edward Schillebeeckx has discussed eight different rational attempts to find a meaning for pain, and he ruefully concludes that we have here "an impenetrable theoretically unreachable mystery." He adds that "human reason does not know what to do with the historical alliance of suffering and evil. Here the human logos, man's rationality, fails. It has no explanation to give." [3] In other words, pain is not a problem that can be logically solved or intelligently explained. He says further that because of the history of human suffering there will always be "human doubt as to whether God is a God of love, and thus whether God exists." Thus, the individual who was led to religious belief because of the puzzle of pain now faces the paradox of the God who allows such suffering.

This presents a genuine difficulty for the believer because he now meets the apparent incompatibility between a good and provident God on the one hand, and the pain and hurt that continue to exist in the world this same God created. Peter Berger notes: "The individual suffering from a tormenting illness, say, or from oppression and exploitation at the hands of fellowmen, desires relief from these misfortunes. But he equally desires to know *why* these misfortunes have come to him in the first place." [4] Even for the unbeliever, who omits God from the equation and thus foregoes this dilemma, suffering persists as an inexplicable phenomenon. The search for meaning is a characteristic quality of human beings, and one is tempted to suggest that the person acts less than human who proclaims the absurdity and meaninglessness of all existence. [5]

On the other hand, one need not be a complete agnostic if she or he gives up the search for an explanation of pain and suffering. A mystery is by definition inexplicable; the divine puzzle simply has no solution attainable by the human mind. Perhaps each generation rediscovers the dilemma of theodicy, and each generation has its share of agnostics and atheists. We should remind ourselves, however, that ancient Hebrew classics like Job and Ecclesiastes had already deeply explored this same juxtaposition of a loving God and a suffering humanity. "They conclude that suffering is so mysterious that it is ultimately meaningless to mere mortals. The point is well made: Judeo-Christianity is solidly grounded in reality and not afraid to admit limitations. For, whatever else suffering may be, it *is* ultimately mysterious, and we shall never understand completely the reason for the cross." [6]

The inability to fathom the puzzle of human suffering need not, then, lead one to embrace atheism or agnosticism. The state of mental uncertainty, whether in a believer or a nonbeliever, may free one to speculate about a world without pain. One might put imagination to work and ask: what would I have done differently if I were the Creator? Any thoughtful man, says Albert Outler, "might well imagine that he could have devised a cosmic operation less replete with frustration, suffering and indignity." [7] This may be a useless exercise but it is the kind of speculation people indulge in when they dream of "what might have been." At the same time, it may be a very frustrating experience because it necessarily implies our powerlessness in altering the past shape of creation and suggests also that the mind of God is inscrutable.

The humble admission that there is no solution to the problem of pain does not in itself satisfy the questing human mind, but it may underline the fact that there are other theological mysteries besides suffering. Believers realize that the transcendent God is wrapped in inexplicable mystery; the human intelligence cannot grasp divinity. When we say, however, that pain is a mystery that does not make sense at the level of human intelligence, we are talking about an experience quite different from the mysteries of religion as such. We have here something that hurts at a personal level of flesh and bones. Pain is not a thesis in theology; it is not an abstract notion; it is not a theoretical question that can be postponed indefinitely. "Pain is a highly subjective sensation and it cannot be seen, felt or denied by any other than the one who reports it. We all know what it is, for it is a near universal experience, and it is almost always a nuisance to everyone concerned." [8] It should be clear then that we *know* pain in a way that we can never know theological mysteries such as the nature of God or of human redemption. As a matter of fact, the question of ignorance and knowledge does not center on the existence or the experience of pain and suffering. It centers on the unanswerable enigma of causality and explanation and meaning: Why do human beings have to suffer? This is the mystery with which the human race has struggled at all times past. We have therefore not unraveled the mystery of pain when we say it is an insoluble problem beyond the grasp of human intelligence.

Acceptance of Suffering

The second approach to human pain and suffering is to accept, even to embrace, these misfortunes in the name of God. Throughout Judeo-Christian history, theologians, mystics and ascetics have asked believers to see a positive aspect in Job or the "suffering servant" or the cross of Christ in relation to their own suffering and pain. Thus Christians should try, even cheerfully, to "offer it up," as the Apostle Peter taught: "Rejoice in so far as you share Christ's suffering, that you may also rejoice and be glad when his glory is revealed." [9] The Judeo-Christian tradition affirms that orthodox theology provides the answer to the question of theodicy. From the specifically Christian point of view "it is crucial that the incarnate God is also the God who suffers." [10] Peter Berger supports this remark with the words of Albert Camus: because "Christ had suffered, and had suffered voluntarily, suffering was no longer unjust and all pain was necessary." [11]

The acceptance of personal pain, whether grudgingly or cheerfully, does not solve the dilemma of theodicy. The paradox remains, but this is one plausible way that people of the Judeo-Christian tradition have in trying to "make sense" out of an otherwise inexplicable phenomenon. Why Job, or the "suffering servant," or Christ is the model of eternal salvation is in itself a profound mystery.[12] There has indeed been a traditional adherence to the positive aspects of human misfortune. Michael Taylor remarks: "From apostolic times Christians have been told and have believed that suffering and death are not without purpose. Christians make sense of life not by closing their eyes to man's anguish, or by wishing it away, but by accepting it and opening the darkness of life to Christ's light."[13] Donald Gelpi goes even further: "The believer who suffers with Christ in faith transforms mere suffering into deepened trust in God and openness to his life-giving Spirit. For faith tested in the crucible of pain is purified by the refusal to test God, even in the midst of personal suffering."[14] Similar affirmations could be proffered from Hebraic and Islamic sources. At the level of daily hospital experience, the great majority (91 percent) of the health professionals we queried were willing to say that "faith in God lessens the fears and anxieties of the suffering person," but a much smaller proportion (39 percent) agreed that "the more religious a person is, the more able he or she is to endure suffering."

The willingness to accept suffering as a means to perfect one's total personality is a hard doctrine for technological man to follow and it probably confounds many conscientious Christians. It proclaims that there is a positive good in suffering and it recalls the rigid and harsh notion that "character is built in adversity." There is no question that ambitious people willingly undergo hardships for the purpose of secular achievement, whether or not their moral character is developed. Perhaps the nonbelieving and areligious stoic can appreciate this kind of attitude, but Christian theologians argue that "those who believe in the providence of a loving God and those who see Christ as a friend as well as a savior will have an entirely different view of suffering." [15] It is the "faith vision" that is said to make the difference. In this view, "pain, suffering, and death disposes for personal transformation." One may even lay down the proposition that suffering can be "an avenue to joy." [16] This peculiar notion that there is joy in suffering, or that pain provides a reason to rejoice, is interpreted by Ladislaus Boros as a kind of transference. Suffering people are srrogates for those who are healthy and pain-free. People who bear their sickness in the light of religious faith, he writes, "give us the chance of living in light, or abandoning ourselves to joy. Someone must bear the world's suffering so that others may have it easier. If you are that one, then thank your Lord every day for being allowed to suffer, for being able to share in his work of redeeming the world. Suffering is election." [17]

In earlier times, even within American culture, it seems to have been a common teaching that the religious person should voluntarily accept the pain that comes in the normal course of living. The reality was, of course, that painkilling drugs were not available, and their production had not evolved into an enormously profitable business. More than that, however, it was thought virtuous that the believer practice self-denial, and even seek to "mortify" himself in taking on further pain and suffering. There was a spiritual value not only in enduring the normal discomfort of the human condition, but also in "doing penance" for one's sins. This is how one gains eternal salvation. Each person has only one lifetime in which to pass the test of trials and tribulations. The patience of Job was the model virtue. Instead of asking why God permits all the misery and suffering in the world, the true believer simply accepts God's will.[18]

From a relatively secular perspective, psychologist Louise Riscalla has written that "suffering is not an enemy or something unpleasant, but an ally in the opportunity to grow into a richer, more healthy individual." She warns, however, against the peculiar "self-indulgence" of readily welcoming pain into one's life. "Religious practices involving indulgence in perpetual penitence and self-mortification are actually forms of masochism in the name of God." Her thesis is that the genuine advantage of suffering is realized when the individual decides to embrace a more spiritual and moral pattern of conduct. "Suffering could be of therapeutic value primarily as a warning that man is not living right and motivate one to correct erroneous ways of living." [19] The willingness to accept pain as a "gift" from God, or as a personal benefit, does not diminish its harsh reality. Whatever one's psychological attitude, this continues to be a world of anguish, misery and tragedy. The traditional pious practices of self-abnegation provide a systematic manner in which believers may learn to live with the enigma of pain.

Rejection of Pain

Even the casual observer of religious attitudes and practices will note that this whole scheme of voluntary mortification has fallen largely into disuse. Partly because of this lessening of interest, the Stauros Association was moved to sponsor the First International Ecumenical Congress on the Meaning of Human Suffering in the spring of 1979, which dealt mainly with the theological, biblical and ascetical aspects of the problem.[20] Religion continues to teach us to accept the disabilities of the human condition, but even religious people are becoming restive about this teaching. A Dutch Protestant pastor of wide experience in the hospital ministry tells us: "Increasingly the right to live and to live happily is regarded as one of the basic rights of men. Hence we are more likely to rebel against suffering and death than to accept them as inevitable constituents of our existence." [21] People in western society are now well aware that much can be done to assuage pain, and that many diseases have been controlled and formerly fatal epidemics have been averted.

The basic experiential fact is that pain is not "nice"; it does not seem an acceptable medium for the attainment of lofty spiritual goals. Bedside nurses have no illusions about the "mystique" of suffering. Their professional function is to alleviate pain and to make their patients as comfortable as possible when pain is unavoidable. In this cultural atmosphere, the only acceptable "value" in pain is that it acts as a warning that something may be seriously "wrong" in the body, which in turn could lead to even more serious suffering.

The widespread attitude of rejection of pain seems to come also now from another and more significant source. This is basically a religious notion, or theological interpretation, that one hears frequently from Pentecostal Christians who insist that "God does not want you to hurt." The popular preacher, Asa Allen, stated this idea most clearly: "It is my firm belief, and this belief is based upon the Scriptures, that God created man healthy and strong, and that God meant for him to continue in that state. And it is also my firm belief that God wants every one of us to prosper and be in health until we fulfill the number of our days." [22] Faith healers proliferated among Protestant Pentecostals in the early twentieth century, and they are now reaching millions of people through the media of radio and television. The most spectacular of the healers is Oral Roberts, who not only recommends physicians to his followers but has also built a large teaching hospital and diagnostic clinic adjacent to his university in Tulsa.[23]

Duquesne University was the site of the beginnings of Pentecostalism among American Catholics in 1968. This charismatic renewal movement was started by lay persons, university professors, who got their early inspiration from Protestant Pentecostal ministers.[24] The special charism of healing is prominently discussed at the renewal prayer meetings, and the intense petition to God for miraculous intervention is most often voiced in separate prayer sessions which occur after the regularly scheduled prayer meetings. In a study of the Catholic charismatic movement we found that more than one-third (37 percent) of the prayer groups had experienced a physical healing among the members.

The most vocal exponent of the healing ministry in the American Catholic Church, until his resignation from the priesthood, was Francis MacNutt, whose books on this subject have become bestsellers. With his wife, he continues to function in the leadership of the Pentecostal movement, which supports the established doctrine that "God wants everyone healed." Sickness is in no way a blessing. One gets the impression that Satan is the source of all suffering and that the demons must be exorcised in removing the curse of illness. "The *basic* source of sickness is the primordial evil which weighs upon man and can only be lifted by a power beyond our human intelligence and activity." [25] A central point in this charismatic philosophy is that Jesus indeed suffered and felt great pain, but had never been afflicted with the curse of sickness.

Faith healers obviously acknowledge the existence of pain, but they reject it as an evil of which God himself disapproves. With a shared belief in the healing power of God and in the spirit of ecumenism, the charismatic followers attend the prayer services of an Agnes Sanford or a Kathryn Kuhlman as well as of a David Du Plessis and a Francis MacNutt. The healers are always careful to disclaim any personal ability to cure the sick. This power to heal is the power of God, who intervenes miraculously and selectively. In other words, not every person is healed, and MacNutt points out that "God's normative will is that people will be healed, unless there are some countervailing reasons." [26] Many times, certainly more often than not, the healing does not take place, and the minister has to provide an explanation as to why God has not heard the prayer for healing. It is an interesting fact that MacNutt lists eleven reasons why the prayer for healing is not answered, but only one of them is the lack of faith in the sick person.

Notes

1 Francis X. Cleary, "Biblical Perspectives on Suffering," *Hospital Progress* 55 (December 1974): 54–58. The universal experience of suffering, injustice, and meaninglessness is termed the common "substructure" of all religions by J. Milton Yinger, "A Comparative Study of the Substructures of Religion," *Journal for the Scientific Study of Religion* 16, no. 1 (March 1977): 67–86.

2 Ladislaus Boros, *Pain and Providence*, trans. Edward Quinn (Baltimore: Helicon, 1966), p. 9.

3 E. Schillebeeckx, "The Mystery of Injustice and the Mystery of Mercy," trans. Michael Fitzpatrick, *Stauros Bulletin*, no. 3 (1975): 11. See also F. J. Buytendijk, *Pain: Its Modes and Functions* (Chicago: University of Chicago Press, 1962), p. 26, "Pain is painful in a double sense, since it is also a puzzle tormenting us."

4 See the helpful sociological insights of Peter Berger, *The Sacred Canopy* (Garden City: Doubleday, 1969), chap. 3, "The Problem of Theodicy," pp. 53–80.

5 The more vocal of critics find their exponent of absurdity in Jean-Paul Sartre. Cf. *Being and Nothingness*, trans. Hazel Barnes (New York: Philosophical Library, 1956).

6 Cleary, "Biblical Perspectives," p. 54.

7 Albert Outler, "God's Providence and the World's Anguish," in *The Mystery of Suffering and Death*, ed. Michael J. Taylor (New York: Alba House, 1973), pp. 3–23.

8 Victor Christopherson, "Sociocultural Correlates of Pain Response," *Social Science* (January 1971): 33–37.

9 1 Peter 4:13. See also Joseph Blenkinsop, "We Rejoice in Our Sufferings," in Taylor, *Mystery of Suffering*, pp. 45–55.

10 Berger, *Sacred Canopy*, p. 76.

11 Albert Camus, *The Rebel* (New York: Vintage, 1956), p. 34.

12 See for example John Hick, *Evil and the God of Love* (New York: Harper & Row, 1966); also Jacques Maritain, *God and the Permission of Evil* (Milwaukee: Bruce, 1966).

13 Taylor, *Mystery of Suffering*, Introduction, p. x.

14 Donald Gelpi, *Charism and Sacrament* (New York: Paulist Press, 1976), p. 90.

15 Kevin D. O'Rourke, "Is Your Health Facility Catholic?" *Hospital Progress* 55 (April 1974): 40–44, 66.

16 Louise Hageman, "Suffering—An Avenue to Joy,"

Humanitas 9, no. 1 (January 1966): 84–96. Charles Davis, before he resigned from the ministry and the church, wrote that "Christians rejoice in suffering because in Christ it meaningfully expresses what men need and long to express." See his article, "Suffering with Christ," *America*, 13 August 1966, p. 157.

17 Boros, *Pain and Providence*, p. 64.

18 See Joseph H. Fichter, "Pastoral Ministry to the Sick, Suffering, and Dying," *Pastoral Life*, xxvii, no. 5 (May 1978): 2–8.

19 Louise Mead Riscalla, "The Therapeutic Value of Suffering," *Journal of the American Society of Psychosomatic Dentistry and Medicine* 20, no. 4 (October 1973): 115–20. See, however, the scientist's strong objection to the notion that "pain is a reaction of defence, a happy warning, which puts us on guard against the dangers of illness, that it is useful, perhaps even necessary." A. Soulairac, "On an Experimental Approach to Pain," in *Pain*, ed. A. Soulairac, J. Cahn, and J. Charpentier (New York: Academic Press, 1968), pp. 3–7.

20 Stauros International Association, with a General Secretariat in Louvain, was organized by the Congregation of the Passion in 1973 "to promote the study of the gospel of Jesus' Passion" and to encourage projects which try to "discover the full dimensions of this mystery at the level of scholarly research." The congress was held at Notre Dame University in April, 1979.

21 Heije Faber, *Pastoral Care in the Modern Hospital*, trans. Hugo de Waal (Philadelphia: Westminster, Press, 1977), p. 49. Ernest Wallwork, "Attitudes in Medical Ethics," in *Nourishing the Humanistic in Medicine*, ed. William Rogers and David Barnard (Pittsburgh: University of Pittsburgh Press, 1979), pp. 125–51, remarks that relief from physical pain "is a particularly urgent moral claim precisely because without such relief there is precious little that one can effectively do or become."

22 Quoted by David Harrell, *All Things are Possible: The Healing and Charismatic Revivals in Modern America* (Bloomington: Indiana University Press, 1975), p. 85.

23 Among his other writings see *The Call* (New York: Doubleday, 1972). See "Oral Roberts' Gift Adds to a Hospital Glut," *Business Week*, 31 October 1977, p. 35.

24 See J. Massyngberde Ford, *Which Way for Catholic Pentecostals?* (New York: Harper & Row, 1976), also Joseph H. Fichter, *The Catholic Cult of the Paraclete* (New York: Sheed and Ward, 1975).

25 Francis MacNutt, *The Power to Heal* (Notre Dame: Ave Maria Press, 1977), p. 129.

26 Francis MacNutt, *Healing* (Notre Dame: Ave Maria Press, 1974), chap. 18, "Eleven Reasons Why People Are Not Healed." See also Mary E. Peterman, *Healing: A Spiritual Adventure* (Philadelphia: Fortress Press, 1974), chap. 5, "What Can I Do To Be Healed?"

Chapter 4

Do Suffering Patients Turn to God?

The dilemma of theodicy involves a relationship with God as well as an attitude toward suffering.[1] Both are realities with which humankind must cope: pain is not banished from the world; neither is God. When people are in physical pain, they seek relief from doctors and nurses and pharmacists, and for the most part they develop great confidence in medical and therapeutic science as a means of "killing pain."[2] People vary in their interpretation of the meaning of suffering: from those who embrace it as a path of redemption to those who see it as a curse that can be removed by the healing power of prayer. Sick patients also differ in the way they relate their pain to God.

Where does God come into the process of pain relief? On the one hand, Jesus is proclaimed the greatest healer, and His followers have always been taught to seek God's help in their suffering and distress. On the other hand, if pain is an inexplicable mystery—as the theologians assert—it would appear that God is remote from the suffering world. In pursuing this question among both patients and health-care professionals, we find that the responses fall into several general categories. First, there are some patients, even dangerously ill ones, who have no interest at all in religion or spirituality, and see no reason for developing such an interest. A second category is that of the true believers, the devoutly religious patients who seek divine assistance, and have been accustomed all their lives to prayerful practices. Thirdly, there are also some patients, bitter after long years of suffering, who actually turn against God and proclaim themselves atheists.

Ignoring God

If secularism is as widespread as many commentators think it is, we must not be surprised that modern people are simply indifferent to God, even when they suffer deep pain or anguish. The secularist has dealt with many of life's problems without paying attention to God and simply continues along the same line when tragedy strikes. Martha Lear's absorbing account of the fatal illness of her physician husband has no reference to God except as an occasional expletive.[3] This casual attitude is clearly evident in Stewart Alsop's story of his struggle with leukemia. On one occasion, "with a certain sense of embarrassment," he entered an Episcopal church near the hospital and tried to recite the Lord's Prayer. "I wish I could say that this strange experience with leukemia has given me profound spiritual insights. But it hasn't. The big bearded reality of my childhood is no longer a reality to me, which was why I felt a faint sense of embarrassment. I have been an agnostic since I was about eighteen. I am an agnostic still." [4] Similarly, Doris Lund tells the dramatic story of her son, Eric, who was afflicted with leukemia at age seventeen and died five years later. During his sickness, he turned for solace, with his mother's approval, to a sexual episode with a sympathetic nurse. Nowhere in the book is there mention of religion, spirituality, God, or prayer in this experience, and no indication that there were chaplains available, or a pastoral care department, at the Sloan Kettering Cancer Center in New York, where Eric was in therapy. Only after his death do we learn that Eric had a friend who was a minister. "There was a memorial service in the church by the River. It was the same Church where Eric had started out to be head counselor in the boys' camp the summer before he died." [5]

The nonbeliever has had no ties to religion and is often from a family which held no membership in a church. Hospital chaplains have frequent contact with patients of this sort: the man or woman who is quite ready to have a friendly chat with the chaplain, to talk about the normal topics of everyday experience, and who shows nothing but a passing curiosity about religious matters. "They are polite and cheerful," says one minister, "and they thank you for visiting them. But they don't know anything about religion and see no reason why they should." Even on their bed of pain when they may be extremely uncomfortable, these people continue to reflect a kind of friendly tolerance that is characteristic of a religiously indifferent society. There is nothing bigoted or hostile in their attitudes.

A deeply spiritual person may be perplexed at the casual manner in which God and religion are dismissed even as death approaches. The parents of Jane Zorza brought her to a hospice to make her last days easier: "The doctor was a deeply religious man, and we had been a little concerned that Jane's atheism might cause problems. There was a priest at the Hospice for those who wanted him. When we arrived, we were asked what Jane's religion was, and when we said 'none,' the subject was never mentioned again." [6] After their daughter died, the parents said they experienced an important change in themselves. "We think far more than we ever did about what really matters in life, about feelings, about the more abiding human values, about people—about people as individuals."

A priest psychiatrist we interviewed told of a patient who said quite calmly, "Well, I have this tumor, and I've thought about death." The priest asked her if the thought of death frightened her. She said: "No, I talked it over with my mother and my family, and I'm satisfied that death is final. There isn't anything afterward." The priest related this incident as a demonstration of the fact that nonbelievers are sometimes able to face death with a calm serenity which is founded neither in opiates nor in religious faith. It may well be that God speaks to individuals in ways that are unfamiliar to the believer, who is sure that God is somehow present to the sick patient, even to the nonreligious one.

This type of patient presents a dilemma to the hospital chaplain, who wants to bring God to sick people. Some of the younger clergy who have had training for the clinical pastoral vocation told us: "You must meet the patient where he is. You do not impose yourself or your religion on him. You stay at his level until he is ready to actualize himself." This seems to mean that the patient who has had no religious experience or knowledge will be forever unable to "actualize" a religious dimension. At the same time, the hospital chaplain is expected to wait for something religious to "happen" to a basically secular and nonreligious person. It appears that pastoral counseling in a conversational vacuum of this kind is completely nonproductive. The chaplain who values psychological procedures over theological content may persuade himself that he shows respect for the spiritual autonomy of the patient. Meanwhile he cheats the patient of the basic privilege to receive God's message of concern and providence.[7]

The religiously indifferent person is sure that he has problems of sickness, and is not aware of problems of religion. The sick person may be anxious, bored, frightened, lonely, and the pastoral visitor may be of great assistance in meeting these moods. Robert Wheelock points out: "The chaplain is especially trained to notice and to address himself to the various feelings and emotions that the patient makes known to him in verbal and nonverbal signs. The modern chaplain is not expected to visit every patient every day. Rather, he is best used in his particular talents when he sees patients who have specific problems and he is able to address himself to these problems." [8] The specific problem for the agnostic is that he has no problem with which the spiritual therapist can grapple.

The particular talents of the pastoral counselor have to be used from a theological perspective; this is what lends both credence and purpose to the chaplain's role.[9] With a more elastic interpretation of that role, one may say that the chaplaincy provides an indirect service to the patient who ignores God and religion. The chaplain takes on a psycholog-

ical task and assumes the role of counselor. In this proce-
dure, then, he is attending to neither a physical nor a
spiritual need, but is attempting to assuage the emotional
needs of the patient. It may well happen that somewhere in
the midst of this psychological counseling the clergyman
will come to the subject of religion and of God's relation to
the sick patient. This may be a circuitous but effective way
of doing the central task of chaplaincy.

Seeking Divine Help

When we asked health-care personnel whether sick patients respond religiously to pain, they most frequently said
that it depends on the religious background of the individual. It is a commonplace generalization that "illness
heightens religious feelings." As Marion Kahn, a medical
social worker, says, "often there is at least a greater preoc-
cupation with religion and perhaps a reassessment of the
place of religion in the life—and death—of the individual." [10] This may be an examination of conscience that
leads to the conclusion that this pain is nothing more than
one deserves. "Some individuals regard illness and suffering as an intrusion God has sent into their lives to punish
them for some past faults or failures." [11] These people feel
guilty and they pray to God to forgive them for past moral
transgressions, real or imagined.

Quite aside from the patient who has feelings of guilt, or
who is convinced that pain is a punishment for sins, many
people have the normal fears and anxieties that accompany
admission to a hospital. Most of the time patients do not
know what is the matter with them or what is going to happen to them. As one nurse told us: "They are really worried
the first time they come in here, especially if they are going
to have an operation. They start saying their prayers, or at
least they start thinking about it." According to Laurel
Copp, a nursing instructor, "some patients stated that suffering, the response to pain, seemed to begin even before
the pain and included many anticipatory fears that sometimes were even more acute than the eventual pain." [12] In

our survey of hospital personnel, we proposed to them the generalization that "faith in God lessens the fears and anxieties of the suffering person." Hardly any respondent disagreed with this statement; only a few were hesitant to answer, but the great majority—nine out of ten—felt that this is true. This high proportion of affirmative answers was the same for all respondents, clergy, nurses, doctors, social workers, for the most pious among them as well as for the least. They may have assumed that most of these suffering patients in church-related hospitals are believers, people who actually have faith in God, and who would be likely to turn to God in the anxieties and fears that accompany their sickness. This is therapeutic only in a secondary sense and does not refer to a diminishment of actual physical pain.

There is much research evidence to support the generalization that the people who turn to God when they are sick are usually also the people who turned to God when they were healthy. Raymond Carey has demonstrated that patients who had lived genuinely religious lives tended to make a better emotional adjustment to the fact that they were terminally ill. He found that those with an "intrinsic religious orientation" exhibited the highest degree of emotional adjustment.[13] This does not exclude the possibility of religious conversion of other patients or the likelihood that a minister of religion may strike the spark of faith in the nonreligious person.

To test further the relationship between pain and religion, we asked the health-care personnel in these hospitals if it is true that "the more religious a person is the more able he or she is to endure suffering." All the respondents to this questionnaire have daily contact with the sick and suffering, and only about four out of ten (39 percent) were ready to answer affirmatively. It is interesting to note that the clergy chaplains were more likely (48 percent) to agree with it than the laywomen hospital nurses (31 percent), who work longer and closer with people in pain. This is, of course, secondhand and subjective information from observers, and it may merely be that the ministers of religion have greater confidence in the strength of religion. Only a minority of these experienced professionals whose task is to take care of the sick were willing to say that strong spiritual faith helps the patient to endure pain, but there have been reports also from patients themselves. The man who agreed to serious medical tests said: "I hope that my submission to these experiments will restore men and women to normal living in years to come .... If they do, I will have aided the scientific advances of man and repaid those who helped me, in the manner which I think God would expect." [14] This patient was a real believer, willing to submit to experimental medical and surgical research. He not only trusted God but prayed that his own suffering might provide medical knowledge of some eventual utility to other suffering people.

While the forms and attitudes of religion have been changing in recent decades, there are still many patients in church-related hospitals who want to continue the prayers and devotions they have known throughout their life, and they rely on them quite naturally when they are confined to the hospital bed. This is an interdenominational phenomenon which we have recognized at a Baptist hospital in New Orleans, a Catholic hospital in Omaha, a Lutheran hospital in Chicago, and a Presbyterian hospital in Albuquerque. Among the younger patients in all of these places, prayer has tended to become less formalized than it had been with their elders, but there is no suggestion that religion is less significant to them.

The two hypotheses offered in the relation of pain to religion test out differently. It seems quite evident that the more religious a person is, or has been during the course of life, the more likely he or she is to turn to God in times of serious illness. The patient who has previously paid little attention to religion will not pray to God. The second hypothesis is that strong religious faith makes it somewhat easier for the patient to endure pain. For the most part, the health professionals in the hospitals we surveyed were not ready to confirm this hypothesis.

Becoming an Atheist

There is some evidence from research that pain may be a hindrance rather than an aid in developing a religious response. This problem seems to be particularly acute with persons who suddenly find themselves in the emergency room of a large city hospital. An experienced chaplain put it this way: "When a person is in crisis, he doesn't have the power to think or reflect about the crisis. The best you can do is to assure the individual that God is there to be of help, but even then you are not sure that you got that idea through to the patient." The person is distraught; pain drives everything else from his mind. Another veteran chaplain said that "alleviating fear is one of the biggest things in the emergency room because people don't know what's in store for them."

We have seen that hospital personnel generally believe that when sick people are anxious and fearful they are strengthened by the consolations of religion. There are instances, however, when the opposite occurs. The immediate effect of intense pain seems to preoccupy patients with themselves and their own troubles in this unhappy situation. The greater the pain, the less likely are such patients to be fresh and alert, able to carry on a conversation with a chaplain, ready to pray and meditate. The Dominican anthropologist, François Lepargneur, argues that "the effects of sickness, far from making it easiser to bring about a spiritual renewal, complicate the difficulty by weakening the capacity for seeing higher values by diminishing the person's interior lucidity." [15]

People who do not believe in the existence of God cannot logically curse God for allowing them to suffer or for visiting pain upon them. People who profess a religious faith, however, may question the providence of God and come to the conclusion that their faith has been misplaced. In other words, severe pain may be a test of religious faith, and a perduring sickness may undermine whatever previous beliefs the patient had. Pastor Faber talks about those who "through suffering lose their faith. They engage in a futile rebellion, they feel cheated, they cannot wrestle through to any meaning in it at all, they begin to complain, they cannot keep up fruitful relationships with their fellows so that there is no chance of consideration for others, of sympathy, of thinking and feeling things through with others; they feel themselves finally alone and cut off." [16]

In so far as we can safely generalize from the terminal therapy recommended by Elisabeth Kubler-Ross and her theory of five stages of dying, we may suggest that the patient is at odds with God in the second stage.[17] Between the initial stage of "denial" and the third stage of "bargaining" the patient goes through a period of hostility and anger. It is questionable whether all, or even most, dying patients experience this sequence of steps. Her theory is built on the assumption that, at least in some instances, the frustrated and helpless person's rage is directed against God. This is supposedly a transitory hostility, after which the individual experiences a period of bargaining with God, then of depression, and finally the fifth stage of acceptance of approaching death. The nurses and social workers at the several hospice programs we visited observed some occasional anger in terminally ill patients, but not in the neat sequence of the Kubler-Ross theory.[18]

Religious believers may be disedified by stories about people who reject God entirely; yet "failures" of this kind can be related by experienced pastors and chaplains. There is the man in a veterans' hospital suffering chronic and intractable pain. The priest chaplain spoke to him of the passion of Christ, the agony and suffering and crucifixion. The patient responded sharply and bitterly: "Don't tell me about your man on the cross. He suffered only a few hours, and then it was all over. I've been in this place more than fifteen years, and never had a day without pain." We do not know whether this military veteran "lost the faith" as a result of sickness and suffering, whether he had never been a religious believer, or whether the very vehemence of his feelings may have been a kind of "negative faith."

Permanent alienation from God is often the case with

persons who are crippled or incurable, although they may not be in constant pain. A certain amount of publicity comes to people who carry on their everyday activities in spite of being paralyzed or in an iron lung or who bravely return from pilgrimages to holy shrines like Lourdes or Fatima or Guadalupe still crippled but with undiminished faith. Apparently these cases are most noteworthy because they are most exceptional. Nurses who work with the permanently disabled report that many of these persons can be helped to "manage their lives" psychologically and emotionally and as far as possible bodily, but they tend to be frustrated in relation to God and religion.

In general, however, we do not have much evidence from our interviews and questionnaires in church-related hospitals concerning sick people who turn away from God in their pain. Some nurses have speculated that the patients are often too sick, and sometimes too polite, to make known their feelings about God. It is generally considered unseemly—if not un-American—to criticize religion and to find fault with God and his ministers. Many secularists and nonbelievers, including physicians, tend to be courteous to the hospital chaplains, even while ignoring the religion which the minister of God represents. In Catholic hospitals, even agnostics tend to speak highly of the "good Sisters."

Notes

1 This chapter is a revision of the article, "Do Suffering Patients Turn to God?" *Hospital Progress* 61, no. 3 (March 1980): 52–55.

2 A vehement though scholarly analysis of "The Killing of Pain" is presented by Ivan Illich, *Medical Nemesis: The Expropriation of Health* (New York: Bantam Books, 1977), pp. 129–50.

3 Martha Weinman Lear, *Heartsounds* (New York: Simon & Schuster, 1980). At the end there was a "sunny memorial service" with a eulogy by a physician and even a "psalm from Corinthians," but with not a rabbi in sight.

4 Stewart Alsop, *Stay of Execution: A Sort of Memoir* (Philadelphia: Lippincott, 1973), p. 149.

5 Doris Lund, *Eric* (Philadelphia: Lippincott, 1974), p. 342.

6 Victor and Rosemary Zorza, "Bringing Humanity to a Daughter's Dying," *Globe and Mail* (Toronto), 2 March 1978, p. 11. We are informed that they are writing a book about their daughter and about the hospice way of dying.

7 For practical insights, see Dennis E. Saylor, *And You Visited Me* (Medford: Morse Press, 1979), chap. 5, "Spiritual Therapy."

8 Robert D. Wheelock, *Health Care Ministries* (St. Louis: Catholic Hospital Association, 1975), p. 46.

9 See the comments of E. S. Golden, "What Influences the Role of the Protestant Chaplain in an Institutional Setting?" *Journal of Pastoral Care* xvi (1962): 218–25.

10 Marion Kahn, "Some Observations on the Role of Religion in Illness," *Social Work* 3 (July 1958): 83–89.

11 Gerald Niklas and Charlotte Stefanics, *Ministry to the Hospitalized* (New York: Paulist Press, 1975), p. 8. See also Dennis E. Saylor, *And You Visited Me* (Medford: Morse Press, 1979), chap. 2, "The Relationship of Sin and Sickness."

12 Laurel A. Copp, "The Spectrum of Suffering," *American Journal of Nursing* 74, no. 3 (March 1974): 491–95.

13 See John Shea, "The Terminally Ill, Religion and the Minister: An Interview with Dr. Raymond G. Carey," *Journal of Pastoral Counseling* 9, no. 1 (Spring-Summer 1974): 63–67.

14 Renée C. Fox, *Experiment Perilous: Physicians and Patients Facing the Unknown* (Glencoe: Free Press, 1959), p. 178.

15 François Lepargneur, "Sickness in a Christian Anthropology," in *The Mystery of Suffering and Death*, ed. Michael J. Taylor (New York: Alba House, 1973), pp. 71–80.

16 Heije Faber, *Pastoral Care in the Modern Hospital* (Philadelphia: Westminster, 1977), p. 43. F. J. Buytendijk, *Pain: Its Modes and Functions* (Chicago: University of Chicago Press, 1962), p. 16, writes of "an immoderate state of algophobia (fear of pain) which is itself an evil."

17 Elisabeth Kubler-Ross, *On Death and Dying* (New York: Macmillan, 1969). See also the earlier article by Cicely Saunders, "The Last Stages of Life," *American Journal of Nursing* 65 (March 1965).

18 See Paul Ramsey, "The Indignity of 'Death with Dignity,'" *Hastings Center Studies* 2 (May 1974): 47–62, and also the criticisms by George Kuykendall, "On Caring for the Dying," *Theology Today* (April 1981), pp. 37–48.

Chapter 5

Religious Response to Sickness

One of the reasons why religion develops an organized existence in the world is that it provides a collective support for human beings who are troubled with misery, anguish, pain, and suffering. Scholars wrestle with the problems of theodicy, and sick people respond in different ways to a provident God, but both healthy intellectuals and sick patients face the basic mystery in pain that is inexplicable. Suffering is part of life, and in some peculiar way it is also intimately connected with the promise of eternal salvation. John McKenzie says that "the gospel does not require us to praise suffering or to affirm that it has a goodness which it does not have. Suffering is part of the human condition, the condition which in biblical language is called a curse."[1] The effort to lift this curse, or at least to lessen its impact, has engaged religious groups even in pre-Christian times, when "resting" places for patients seeking medical treatment were provided under religious auspices in Greece, Egypt, Babylonia, and India.[2] The religious dimension of human crises in suffering and sickness seemed always to arouse some vague theological speculations about the meaning of death. It forces the attention of the individual patient to the immediate response to pain as well as to a personal relation with God. At the level of everyday behavior, we may ask how this personal encounter with pain is translated to a social concern of the religious collectivity. As Dominican theologian Thomas O'Meara remarks: "In health-ministry we go beyond what Christianity says about death and face the question: What does Christianity *do* about illness?"[3]

66

Comfort the Afflicted

Every Christian probably knows that there is no record of Jesus ever being sick, and certainly knows that Jesus is often described as healing the afflicted. According to Mark, he promised that believers would be given certain signs of power: "They will place their hands on the sick, and they will get well." [4] He wanted his followers to have compassion for those in pain. Luke tells us that he called the twelve disciples together and "gave them power and authority to drive out all demons and to cure diseases. Then he sent them out to preach the Kingdom of God and to heal the sick." [5] The "good news" of salvation intimately connects preaching and healing. The example of the compassionate Christ has always been held up for imitation. In the early church, and during the centuries since then, all Christians have been reminded of their obligation in love to be concerned about the welfare of others. In the young Christian communities, special attention was paid to those who needed help: the sick, the widowed, the orphaned. Religious believers heeded the Pauline counsel: "If one member suffer anything, all the members suffer with it, or if one member glories, all the members rejoice with it. Now you are the body of Christ, member for member." [6]

The gift of miraculous healing seems to have been limited to relatively few Christians although, as we have noted, it has been recently emphasized anew among Pentecostals and charismatics. The corporal works of mercy, however, which include the care of sick people, were incumbent on all believers in Jesus. Historically, however, there soon developed a more direct and specialized care of the sick in the ministrations by deacons and deaconesses. It appears that the role of the deaconess included, among other duties, "ministry of nursing service to the sick women at whose homes she regularly visited." [7] Medical treatment and nursing care have always been associated with religious ministry, but the ministry of medicine seems to have been limited to relatively few patients, while nursing reached out to a large population of sufferers.

In principle, Christian love was all-embracing, ideally reaching out to anyone who was sick and suffering, and especially to the poor and needy, who had no one else to care for them. Compared to pre-Christian times, writes C. M. Frank: "Care of the sick underwent an important change. Essentially, Christians enlarged nursing service, making it available to all persons in need regardless of creed or social position, distinguished it from medical practice, gave it some organization, and infused into it the virtue of compassion." [8] What happened then was the development of a nursing ministry among Christians who felt that they had a special vocation to care for the sick. The point emphasized here is that historically the primary motivation for taking care of people in pain was religious. It was for spiritual reasons, for the love of God and in imitation of Christ, that the early Christians organized their nursing ministry. Thomas Szasz even suggests that the function of medicine and religion "have a common origin in the ancient role of the healer (e.g., Jesus Christ.)" [9] The early Christians were drawn exclusively at first to the indigent sick people in the community, who had no one to care for them and who could not afford the services of whatever physicians there were available. Sick people who could afford to pay for medical doctors had the physician visit them at home.

The concept of hospital care for the indigent poor had its Christian origin and development in the diaconate, and gradually the deacons performed more and more the duties of hospital workers and nurses.[10] There were also surely other deaconesses besides the Phoebe mentioned by Saint Paul. The first person to teach the art of nursing is said to have been Paula, a disciple of Saint Jerome. We are told also that a wealthy Christian woman, Fabiola, opened the first Roman institution for the care of the sick. Ivan Illich remarks that hospitals "appeared under Christian auspices in late antiquity as dormitories for travelers, vagrants, and derelicts." [11] Christian charity was pointed at the poor and the needy. When the monasteries developed written constitutions, like the rule of Saint Benedict, they made provision for infirmarians. "Before and above all things, care must be taken of the sick that they be served in very truth as Christ is served." [12]

Growth of Hospitals

The development of the monastic system in western society was conducive to the successful establishment of hospitals under religious auspices. Judaism and Islam also taught that care of the sick and the poor are spiritual obligations because human life is a basic value. Christianity as an institutionalized religion, however, "provided the doctrinal and organizational basis for hospital staffs," so that "for many centuries, European hospitals were run by the church or by associations of laymen affiliated with the church, and they were staffed by nuns. For much of their history they were custodial institutions, where sick and dying people were maintained and given religious guidance." [13] A number of religious orders specifically devoted to nursing were formed according to the monastic rules of Saint Augustine, like the religious Sisters who nursed the sick at the famous Hotel-Dieu in Paris. [14]

While the nursing profession is most commonly thought of as an occupation for women, with Florence Nightingale as the popular British patroness, it was also historically associated with the Knights Hospitallers of Saint John of Jerusalem and the Knights of Saint Lazarus. [15] Saint Camillus de Lellis was proclaimed by Pope Pius XI to be the Patron of Nurses, and his name has been given to the journal of the National Association of Catholic Chaplains. [16] The Alexian Brothers are probably the best known among the male religious orders devoted to hospitals and health care. They were first officially recognized by the church in 1377, and in the United States they operate general hospitals in Chicago, Newark, Saint Louis, and San Francisco. Nevertheless, the great majority of American hospital nurses are female. Protestant deaconesses and Catholic nuns continued to work in hospitals and in the process of secularization helped to develop a new occupation of trained lay nurses toward the end of the nineteenth century. In 1978 the annual survey by the American Hospital Association listed 6,039 short-term general hospitals, of which approximately one-seventh (13.9 percent) were church-related. By far the great majority of the church-related general hospitals (636 out of 838) were conducted under Catholic auspices.[17]

Like other social roles and occupational programs, the corporal works of mercy have become specialized and professionalized in modern technological society. Even the terminology has changed. What had obviously been known as sick care over the centuries is now generally called "health care," or even "medical care," although in many instances the patient needs the nurse more than the medical doctor. The large modern hospital centers its attention on sick patients, but this attention is in many instances a means to two other objectives: maintenance of a medical research laboratory and a clinical training program for students in medical schools. The manner in which the modern hospital relates to the community which it serves has also drastically changed. It maintains emergency rooms, outpatient departments, and specialized clinics, and through these facilities it becomes the health-care center for the entire community. Physicians seldom make "house calls," and now generally expect patients to come to their office, or they instruct the sicker people to meet them in the hospital. We were told repeatedly that more than 80 percent of the patients who come to the emergency room are in need of medical attention but do not need a hospital. It is almost as though the whole system were geared to the convenience of the medical profession. And indeed it has been suggested that "private physicians frequently treat the public, both in the hospital and in their offices, with as uncaring an attitude as is displayed within the hospitals by some hospital personnel." [18]

All public hospitals, as well as the voluntary, nonprofit hospitals, are now seen as the normal locus for sick people.

What was once a moral precept, obeyed by religious believers, has now become an accepted moral duty of the
larger community. Health care and social welfare have become institutionalized as a collective obligation. Most citizens in our society admit that sick people have a right to
financial, or welfare, support. It seems important to repeat
that in the view of the Christian community this human
right of the sick and the poor was met in the Christian hospital. "It was originally not an institution for diagnosis,
treatment and nursing, which would be the modern definition of a hospital, but rather a place in which works of mercy
and compassion could be performed." [19] Compassion for
the poor in the name of Christ has now become compassion
for the sick regardless of their socioeconomic status.

Has the original and historical religious motivation dis-
appeared from the contemporary care of the sick? Has the
high spirituality which was said to characterize the ministry
to the suffering poor now been replaced by the specialized
talent of trained technicians? In practicing the corporal
works of mercy and in comforting the afflicted, the founders
of church-related hospitals were giving a faith response to
human suffering which went beyond the medical expertise
and professional performance of nurses and doctors. Since
this is the case, writes O'Meara, "it is all the more astonish-
ing if they have forgotten or neglected the religious dimension of human life, the climactic position of illness and care
in human religion." [20]

A particularly deep concern for the likely decline of the
religious spirit in the hospital ministry among Roman
Catholics has been expressed at two levels: one is the fact
that fewer religious Sisters are available for hospital duty,
and the other is in the closing of many Catholic schools of
nursing where the principles of spiritual ministry had been
inculcated. This double concern seems to be predicated on
a negative judgment of the spirituality of lay people. Edmund Pellegrino, however, suggests that the religious dimensions of health care can be preserved and promoted by
lay persons. "Protestant colleagues have operated hospitals

dedicated to Christian principles with laymen in key management positions. No Catholic who has visited such hospitals should be presumptuous enough to deny the care provided is less Christian than that provided in a Catholic hospital." [21] As chairman of the Institute on Human Values in Medicine, he also wrote: "All humans must take a stand in respect to the transcendental. All make some act of belief or unbelief. Whatever that act may be, the reality of religion for humankind, especially for the sick, is undeniable." [22]

Spirituality Essential

The question arises, of course, whether modern American health care has lessened its spiritual motivation even in the church-related facilities. In this instance, we are inquiring about the religiosity of the hospital personnel, rather than the spiritual response to pain on the part of patients. It seemed useful, then, to ask the respondents to this survey whether they agree with the statement that "you can't be a good health professional unless you have a spiritual perspective on life." More than three-quarters (78 percent) of them were in agreement. The hospital chaplains, both male and female were highest proportionately in their insistence on the importance of the spiritual perspective, as were the religious Sisters of this study. This proportion of agreement declines to seven out of ten of the medical personnel—physicians 68 percent and nurses 73 percent—and this seems to relate to the personal religiosity of the respondent. The dissenting minority among the physicians and surgeons admit that they are personally "not very" or "hardly at all" religious, even though all of them claim some affiliation with an organized religion.

The majority of respondents in these church-related hospitals are saying that spirituality is necessary, not just helpful, in dealing with the sick. In other words, there is seen here a need to go beyond the physiological and psychological aspects of health care. The materialist, the secularist, the unbeliever is then seen as one who is inadequate to deal with the problems of sickness and pain. The noted physician, Paul Tournier, goes even further than this. He declares: "One cannot tend the body without tending the mind and the spirit. There is no physical reform possible without moral reform. And there is no moral reform without spiritual renewal." [23] The health-care personnel seem in agreement that the lack of a spiritual orientation is a professional deficiency; yet there are arguments to the effect that excellent medical attention can be provided by some people who claim to be agnostics, or even atheists. We are speaking here, of course, about attitudes of preference— what respondents think ought to be—in the character of hospital staff and medical professionals. There is also a minority among the hospital nurses of this study who are not ready to insist that a spiritual perspective is necessary in nursing. We cannot say that the nonbeliever's care of the sick is less competent and less devoted than that of the religiously believing nurse. The fact is that the bedside nurse—whatever her religious orientation—spends more time, and is in closer contact, with the patient than either the physician or the chaplain. It is our impression from interviews and observation that most nurses are very sensitive to the spiritual needs of their patients. Textbooks used in nursing schools usually devote a chapter to this aspect of health care,[24] while the excellent volume by Sharon Fish and Judith Shelley points out the spiritual needs of both patients and nurses as expressed in the professional role of nursing.[25]

Besides the general question about the need for a spiritual perspective among health-care professionals, we asked them whether they considered their own work at the hospital as a spiritual ministry to the sick, and whether they deemed this essential, occasional, or peripheral. It is to be expected that the priests and religious Sisters were almost unanimous in saying that whatever they were doing at the hospital was essentially a spiritual ministry. About seven out of ten of the laywomen nurses saw spiritual ministry as essential to their work, but the proportion of physicians with this response dropped below 60 percent. A significant minority (18 percent) of doctors say that if there is a spiritual ministry involved in health care, it is at best only peripheral to their own work at the hospital. Even if some of the medical practitioners tend to avoid this question, they are probably ready to accept Samuel Mines's generalization: "Today's practicing physician does not underestimate the power of faith, suggestion, psychology, tender loving care, or whatever you wish to call it. He knows how large a share it plays in any case. In the treatment of pain it plays, perhaps a major part." [26] John Stoeckle, physician and clinic director at Massachusetts General, says, "the acts of medical practice are rarely curative." The technical expertise is not central. "As acts of 'doctoring,' all the medical tasks contain human dimensions; in each, the *doctor-patient relation,* not technology, is central." [27]

There is an interesting contrast in these answers to the question of spiritual dimensions of health care. All the respondents were more likely to say that there ought to be spirituality among hospital professionals than to say that they themselves were involved in a spiritual ministry to sick people. Perhaps this is the typical difference between theory and practice, or it may be that ideals are always higher than the implementation of ideals. Perhaps along these lines they were also modestly admitting that they do not fully adhere to the highest description of the good health professional, more willing to say that they are spiritually deficient than that they have any shortcomings in their medical competence.

Holistic Approach

The medical specialist of every kind is prestigious and successful and is in no danger of being replaced by nonspecialists in the foreseeable future. More than three-quarters of all American physicians are medical or surgical specialists, experts in treating only one part of the body or only one aspect of a complicated disease.[28] The shortage of generalists, or family doctors, has become acute at the level of primary health care, and these are the physicians who are most likely to have a holistic approach to medical practice. In recent years, much has been said and written about the holistic patient who is treated as a *whole* human being, not only as a physical entity but also as a psychological, social, and spiritual being. The sick person must not be dealt with segmentally, separately by medicine and by religion. Again, according to Paul Tournier: "We may not say that scientific treatment is the doctor's province, and the cure of the soul the theologian's. To say this would be to condemn both doctors and theologians to see, each of them, but one half of reality." [29]

Not only is the sick patient to be thought of as a whole person, but one may insist that the hospital team and all its members should be holistically oriented. As a logical corollary to the notion that all health professionals should be well-balanced and whole persons who include spirituality in their life-style and philosophy, there should obviously be a similar "wholeness" in the hospital team that cares for the patient. Whether or not one speaks of cooperative teamwork among all the hospital personnel, it is clear that the skills of different specialists and professionals are generally brought to bear on each case.[30] This philosophy is witnessed in those hospitals that attempt to develop themselves as a total therapeutic community, in which everyone working at the hospital at whatever level is concerned about the care of patients. Competent and humane hospital administrators insist on the maintenance of this "caring environment." [31]

The suggestion is sometimes made that only the chaplain can approach the sick person as a whole human being. Irving Rosen argues that the minister should be included "as an *integral* rather than a peripheral part of the health team, a role he is far from fulfilling at this time. With the prevailing enormous amount of psychiatric and psychosomatic disorder for which we have no special medical cures, we should turn for help to specialists in 'the whole person.' " [32] The implication here is that doctors and nurses do not, and perhaps cannot, take care of the "whole" sick person, and that only the pastoral minister, or hospital chaplain, has a holistic approach to the sufferer. One may question also whether the religious practitioner should be called in only for those disorders, psychiatric and psychosomatic, for which there are no specific medical cures. In short, it should be affirmed that the so-called spiritual dimension is present in the health care of all patients, whatever their form of illness. One of the most frequent responses we got when we asked about religion for the sick person was that "it depends on whether the patient is religious." The assumption in this case is that the patient is the only one who has to be holistic, aware of the spiritual as well as the physical and psychological aspects of sickness.

The intent of our question focused on the health professionals themselves when we asked respondents whether they agree with the statement that "the holistic approach in modern health care has to include spiritual ministration to patients." In other words, we wanted to know if they thought that spiritual care is an ingredient of health care. Nine out of ten of all respondents, including physicians, nurses, and social workers, answered in the affirmative.[33] What they seemed to be saying is that the religious perspective of the interdisciplinary health team should be accommodated to the religious perspective of the person in pain. We may take this to mean also that the pastoral-care professional is not to be the only team member to provide spiritual ministry. Everyone working in the hospital is supposed to have a full spiritual perspective on life. The newer "Wholistic Health Centers" exist outside of hospitals and sometimes at a church or parish location. A physician at one of them explained: "Along with the pastoral counselor and nurse, I struggle to find a way that we can effectively and smoothly minister to people who are in pain, in need, who are concerned about their health. It's a startling process to try to get people of two disciplines, counseling and medicine, to work together on an equal footing, but that's what we're struggling to do." [34]

The holistic method is pointed at the goal of healing, helping the person "get better," rather than at the spiritual task of bringing God to the sick person. We are not speaking here of healing some sickness of the soul while the physical aspect of sickness is taken care of otherwise. Holism is a total perspective which assumes that "getting better" cannot be attributed to any single ministration. "Physicians are wont to say that the good doctor does not heal by anything that he does or medicine he prescribes, but rather tries to establish conditions in which the healing forces of nature can do their work. This is true, and the corollary is that the expert counselor, minister, psychiatrist, psychologist, or friend does not offer a single prescription for health or wholeness." [35] The religious dimension is expected to suffuse the total lives of all people, whether they are sick or well. The assumption is, of course, that human beings are by nature something more than material objects, that the spiritual aspect is present whether or not a person recognizes it, or even if one fails to be receptive to meditations about God and religion. There is in the holistic approach "a conviction that one's faith and outlook on life are integral to the health and healing of our body. If health care fails to deal with the spiritual dimension, the patient is not being treated as a whole person." [36]

Purveyors of Religion

In a culture which tends to emphasize the specialization of occupational roles as well as the private nature of religion, one might expect that only trained religious professionals would perform the role of spiritual ministry for people in pain. This, however, is not the general expectation in the church-related hospitals we surveyed. We asked the respondents if they agree that "in the hospital setting no one but a clergyman should talk religion to the patient." Almost unanimously, everyone who gave an opinion disagreed with this statement—ministers, Sisters, nurses, social workers, physicians, administrators. This finding corresponds, of course, with the generalization of the holistic approach: just as religion should not be compartmentalized in the personality of the patients, it should not become a specific and separate role of the pastor or minister. Ideally, everybody in the hospital should be ready to talk religion to the sick people. Spirituality belongs to everybody. This is a reflection of the generalization that religion is an intrinsic and pervading presence throughout professional health care.

More directly to the medically trained people, we asked whether physicians and nurses should be "expected to talk about God with their patients." We were obviously not asking them to replace the clergy in health care, or the chaplains to replace them.[37] Here again, the great majority of all respondents—nine out of ten nurses and eight out of ten physicians—opined that such religious talk is appropriate for them in dealing with the sick. There is no question then that these health professionals in church-related hospitals want everybody to bring God to their patients. They clearly express the ideals of traditional Judeo-Christian ministry to the sick. A nationally recognized hospital administrator argues that church-sponsored health facilities function primarily to advance the quality of human life motivated by distinctive religious values. Communicating the philosophy of religious service to all personnel is a more important part of the apostolate of the church-related hospital than is the direct provision of health care.[38] An even more dramatic challenge was issued by Jerome Wilkerson, who advocated that the staff of these hospitals should focus primary attention on the spiritual works of mercy rather than on the corporal works of mercy.[39]

Several of the interviewees in this study discussed the concept of the hospital as a total healing community where all the people involved in the hospital, from janitors to administrators to head surgeons, would be ministering to the sick and to each other. Every person there was to be responsible for the pastoral care of everyone. As Rex Knowles writes: "We are called to exercise a therapeutic role, one which calls for deep commitment to and deep involvement in common human concerns. This involvement, at its core, can best be referred to as Christian presence—a true presence and availability to others which proceeds from the wholeness so freely given to us and which, as it is shared, becomes the vehicle through which effective healing flows. We have been touched, and it is our responsibility to touch others." [40] The full-time personnel in pastoral-care departments often stressed the importance of "religious presence" in their work. One chaplain had this to say: "The way that I'm different from everybody else in this hospital is that my main job is to *be* with the patients. That's the thing I'm getting paid for. Everybody else who comes in the sick room has to *do* something to or for the patient. All I have to do is to be there." Another minister remarked that this is a significant change from previous patterns of hospital chaplaincy when the chaplain felt that he had to visit every patient every day. "Now I work on the principle that religious needs are not the same for everybody. Some need more attention than others. I stay longer with them."

Nurses are "present" to the patient for longer periods of time than are any of the other hospital personnel. Like other members of the staff, they agree that "God talk" and religious topics need not be restricted to the pastoral personnel, but in our interviews with them they tended to downplay their own ability to converse spiritually with patients. One experienced nurse told us: "I wish I were more able to talk religion and know what to say about God. I think that most of the time I am being spiritual and I'm bringing God to my patients just by doing my job right and by treating them with tender loving care. Sometimes just keeping your patience with crabby sick people is the same as practicing Christlike virtue." In many instances, the nurses seemed to be purveyors of religion by example rather than by speech. And it may very well be that in the long run the practice of Christian virtue conveys a more effective message than conversation and preaching.

Theoretically and ideally the spiritual dimension of health care recalls the original religious motivation for both the personal and organized care of people in pain. As we noted earlier, in the first Christian communities and in the early years of hospitals the whole person was taken care of with physical and bodily relief to the extent that knowledge and techniques were available, but with special concern for spiritual welfare. On the modern hospital scene, the development of specific and exclusive professional roles has tended to obscure this holistic concept. There still remains, however, among the personnel of church-related hospitals a conviction that they should all be responsible purveyors of religion.

Notes

1 John L. McKenzie, "The Son of Man Must Suffer," in *The Mystery of Suffering and Death*, ed. Michael Taylor (New York: Alba House, 1973), pp. 31–44.

2 *Encylopaedia Britannica*, vol. 8 (1974), W. Douglas Piercey "Hospital," pp. 1114–17.

3 Thomas O'Meara, "Christian Ministry and Heath Service," in *The Mission of Healing*, ed. Kevin O'Rourke (St. Louis: Catholic Hospital Association, 1974), pp. 40–47. See also Frederick C. Depp, "Jesus Our Healing Savior and the Sociology of Health," in *A Reader in Sociology: Christian Perspectives*, ed. Charles De Santo, Calvin Redekop, and William L. Smith-Hinds (Scottdale: Herald Press, 1980), pp. 643–58.

4 Mark 16:17–18. This scriptural promise, together with evangelization and the expulsion of demons, is central to Pentecostal groups. See, for example, Bernard Martin, *The Healing Ministry in the Church* (Richmond: Knox Press, 1961). Also Morton T. Kelsey, *Healing and Christianity: In Ancient Thought and Modern Times* (New York, Harper & Row, 1973).

5 Luke 9:1–3. The tradition persists that the evangelist Luke was "our most dear physician," mentioned in Paul's letter to the Col. 4:14

6 I Cor. 12:26–27

7 See Peter Hünermann, "Conclusions Regarding the Female Deaconate," *Theological Studies* 36 (January 1975): 325–33.

8 *New Catholic Encyclopedia*, vol. 10 (1967), C. M. Frank, "History of Nursing," pp. 580–85. See also C. M. Frank, *Foundations of Nursing* (Philadelphia: Saunders, 1959).

9 Thomas S. Szasz, *Pain and Pleasure: A Study of Bodily Feel-*

ings (New York: Basic Books, 1957), p. 68. See also Peter Berger, *Pyramids of Sacrifice* (New York: Basic Books, 1974).

10 See Edward P. Echlin, "Deacons' Golden Age," *Worship* 45 (January 1971): 37–46.

11 Ivan Illich, *Medical Nemesis: The Expropriation of Health* (New York: Bantam Books, 1977), p. 152. In the late Middle Ages, he says, they were "charitable institutions for the custody of the destitute," who died there because "nobody went to a hospital to restore his health."

12 Cited in Frank, "History of Nursing," p. 580.

13 *International Encyclopedia of the Social Sciences*, vol. 10 (1968), William Glaser, "Medical Care: Social Aspects," pp. 93–99. See also George Rosen, "The Hospital: Historical Sociology of a Community Institution," in *The Hospital in Modern Society*, ed. Eliot Freidson (New York: Free Press, 1963), pp. 1–36.

14 See *New Catholic Encyclopedia*, vol. 7 (1967), L. Butler, "Hospitallers and Hospital Sisters," pp. 155–58.

15 See the brief historical sketch by Dennis G. Murphy, *They Did Not Pass By* (New York: Longmans Green, 1956), chap. 4, "The Male Nurse."

16 *Camillian* is a quarterly journal published in St. Louis by the National Association of Catholic Chaplains.

17 We exclude from this study the church-related sanatoria and special hospitals which numbered 86 in 1980 with 539,162 patients. In 1960 they were more numerous (137) but with fewer patients (209,686).

18 Joseph Bean and Rene Laliberty, *Decentralizing Hospital Management* (Reading: Addison-Wesley, 1980), p. 2.

19 Heije Faber, *Pastoral Care in the Modern Hospital* (Philadelphia: Westminster, 1977), p. 6. See also Mary Risley, *House of Healing—The Story of the Hospital* (Garden City: Doubleday, 1961).

20 Thomas F. O'Meara, "Health Care Amid Religion and Revelation," *Hospital Progress* 59 (February 1978): 68–72. See also Joseph H. Fichter, "Spiritual Dimensions of Health Care," *Camillian* 18, no. 3 (Fall 1979): 25–31.

21 Edmund Pellegrino, "The Catholic Hospital: Options for Survival," *Hospital Progress* 56 (February 1975): 42, 52.

22 Edmund Pellegrino, Foreword, in *Medicine and Religion: Strategies for Care*, ed. Donald W. Shriver (Pittsburgh: University of Pittsburgh Press, 1980).

23 Paul Tournier, *The Healing Person* (New York: Harper & Row, 1965), p. 63.

24 See, for example, Beverly Witter Du Gas, *Introduction to Patient Care: A Comprehensive Approach to Nursing* (Philadelphia: Saunders, 1977), chap. 14, "Spiritual Needs."

25 See Sharon Fish and Judith Shelley, *Spiritual Care: The Nurse's Role* (Downers Grove: Intervarsity Press, 1978), "The Nurse's Personal Spiritual Resources," pp. 133–245

26 Samuel Mines, *The Conquest of Pain* (New York: Grosset & Dunlap, 1974), p. 51.

27 John D. Stoeckle, "The Tasks of Care: Humanistic Dimensions of Medical Education," in *Nourishing the Humanistic in Medicine*, ed. William Rogers and David Barnard (Pittsburgh: University of Pittsburgh Press, 1979), 263–75.

28 In 1976 only 17 percent of physicians in patient care were general practitioners. See U.S. Bureau of the Census, *Statistical Abstract of the United States*, 1978, p. 106. Harsh comments are made by Ivan Illich about medical specialists. "By gaining the right to self-evaluation according to special criteria that fit its own view of reality, each new specialty generates for society at large a new impediment to evaluating what its work actually contributes to the health of patients. *Medical Nemesis*, p. 243.

29 Paul Tournier, *A Doctor's Casebook*, trans. Edwin Hudson (New York: Harper & Row, 1960), p. 35.

30 See the enthusiastic account by Robert M. Cunningham, *The Wholistic Health Centers: A New Direction in Health Care* (Battle Creek: Kellogg Foundation, 1977).

31 The management point of view is analyzed by Joseph Bean and Rene Laliberty, *Decentralizing Hospital Management* (Reading: Addison-Wesley, 1980), chap. 1, "Maintaining A Caring Environment."

32 Irving Rosen, "Some Contributions of Religion to Mental and Physical Health," *Religion and Health* 13, no. 4 (October 1974): 289–94.

33 Robert D. Wheelock, "Is Pastoral Care Health Care?" *Hospital Progress* 56 (May 1975): 38, 40, is an answer to the charge that pastoral care is simply duplicating the task of medical social workers.

34 Quoted by Donald A. Tubesing, *Wholistic Health* (New York: Human Science Press, 1979), p. 134. The spelling of "wholistic" is considered a barbarism by scientists who accept the theory of holism.

35 Harry C. Meserve, "Religion's Contribution to Health," *Journal of Religion and Health* 13, no. 1 (January 1974): 3–5.
36 Tubesing, *Wholistic Health*, p. 158. This conviction is expressed also by Dale Dobson, "A Holistic Concept of Illness," in *Pastoral Care in Health Facilities*, ed. Ward A. Knights (St. Louis: Catholic Hospital Association, 1977), pp. 1–3.
37 See the comments of Fish and Shelley, *Spiritual Care*, chap. 8, "Referral to the Clergy." Also Dennis E. Saylor, *And You Visited Me* (Medford: Morse Press, 1979), chap. 9, "The Pastoral Counselor and the Hospital Staff."
38 Sr. Mary Brigh, O.S.F., "Purpose and Need of Church-Sponsored Health Facilities," *Hospital Progress* 49 (September 1968): 59–60.
39 Jerome Wilkerson, "Aggiornamento: Dedication of Religious in Maintaining Catholic Hospitals," *Hospital Progress* 46 (July 1965): 75–77.
40 Rex Knowles, "Christian Presence," in *Pastoral Care in Health Facilities*, ed. Ward A. Knights (St. Louis: Catholic Hospital Association, 1977), pp. 112–14.

Chapter 6
Spirituality in Practice

The conventional wisdom among people involved in health care is a recognition of a continuing trend toward secularization. The central importance of religion for the establishment and maintenance of hospitals has decreased while medical science and technology have grown in importance. "In modern times," writes Pastor Dennis Saylor: "medicine has divorced itself from religion completely and instead has allied itself to scientific methodology. Whereas hospitals in the past were mainly established as the result of religious motivation, the modern medical center has a large laboratory and a small chapel." [1] The central thrust of this study is to test that generalization as exhibited in the spiritual behavior of health professionals in church-related hospitals.

The large number of hospitals that were started by churches attracted, at least in the beginning, health professionals who shared the same faith. Catholic hospitals were staffed mainly by Catholics, Baptist hospitals by Baptists, Methodist hospitals by Methodists, and so it was also in the other denominational institutions. Proportions by denominational affiliation vary widely depending upon the region of the country and religious affiliation of the population, as well as the availability of trained health professionals. For example, in the Catholic hospitals studied, 30 percent of the nurses and medical doctors are not adherents of Catholicism. Nevertheless, the great majority (86 percent) consider themselves religious. They are believers and they agree that religion must be integrated into the multidisciplinary ministry to the sick.

In the area of religious beliefs and attitudes, we find a

consistently higher level of response from the church professionals, ministers, chaplains, religious Sisters. It is expected then that in the spiritual practice of their ministry they would perform according to their high ideals. The fact is, however, that the therapeutic community of the hospital includes increasing numbers of lay people. Joseph Dolan suggests that "the laity in ministry fulfill their baptismal and confirmation promises to love God and neighbor and to reach out to the suffering Jesus in the person of their neighbors. Ministry must involve all Christians—priests, religious, and laity joined in prayer, under the guidance of the Spirit." [2]

Personal Spirituality

We have no direct measure of the personal piety or religious devotion of the respondents to this study. We did ask them to what degree they consider themselves religious, and only 3 percent answered "not very" or "hardly at all." The great majority (88 percent) of all respondents were Roman Catholics, and less than 1 percent reported no affiliation to an organized religion. Aside from the clergy and religious Sisters, about 70 percent of the lay personnel were Catholics. As we have already seen, the great majority of them felt that professionals in health care should have a spiritual perspective on life, and also that the work they do at the hospital should be considered a form of spiritual ministry. [3]

We find also that in actual practice they do bring some aspects of religion into their daily tasks. We asked them, for example, whether they "pray for God's guidance" as they go about their daily work with the sick, and more than nine out of ten answered affirmatively. This is an obvious expression of faith, an admission of dependence on divine providence, and a confidence in the power of prayer. [4] If health care is a total spiritual ministry, one may expect that the people involved in it—at least the priests and Sisters—would be more than normally spiritual. We did not ask about the intensity and frequency of prayer, but we may assume that the lay persons among them are probably similar in this regard to other religious believers.

It is probably true that the social workers, nurses, or physicians tend to be spiritually influenced by daily contact with sickness to the degree that they are persons of faith.[5] This is quite clearly the case with the sick patient. Research evidence indicates that in most instances the religious reaction to pain depends on the patient's own religiosity, that is, previous steadfast adherence to spiritual beliefs and practices. We asked this question now of the health-care professionals themselves. Does the daily experience with sick people bring them "close to God"? All of the clergy and women religious answered in the affirmative, as did eight out of ten of the lay persons. It appears that the presence of pain and misery has a spiritual value for the hospital personnel as well as for the suffering patient.

What is said in reference to the sick person can probably be said also about those who minister to the sick. "Every minister knows that there can be a powerful interaction between a man's faith and his illness." [6] We pursued this matter further by asking the same question from a negative perspective. To what extent would they agree to the statement "the suffering I see every day weakens my faith"? The proportional responses are fairly similar to those given to the previous statement on whether or not contact with people in pain brings them closer to God. Here again, chaplains and religious Sisters are unanimous in denying that their faith in God is weakened in the face of suffering, and almost nine out of ten (87 percent) of the others give the same answer.

We were told by some interviewees that their faith was strengthened by contact with the sick and suffering, and by others that strong religious faith is needed to overcome the emotional stress of the hospital ministry. One experienced nurse said that "when you are with a person in pain, it's very difficult for you not to feel the same helplessness, hopelessness, perhaps frustration, unless you bring to the situation something of yourself, your own philosophy, and really your own spiritual faith." None of the women we interviewed revealed the stereotype of the cold, indifferent, and emotionless nurse.[7] What we heard from them rather was that "when the patient hurts, you hurt a little; when he dies, you die a little. I don't think I could stand it if I did not have my faith in God."

Medical doctors generally seem reluctant to admit anything but an objective and "scientific" reaction to patients in pain. Occasionally, however, one finds a physician or surgeon who realizes the stressful situation involved in dealing with suffering patients. He also is often in need of spiritual sustenance. As one medical doctor remarked: "I, too, need spiritual consultation to do my work better. There is an opportunity for dialogue that makes the clergyman aware that physicians are quite human too—that they get tired, make mistakes in judgment, and often in the loneliness of their profession need spiritual help to fill the void." [8] A more specific manifestation of personal spirituality lies in the practice of prayer. We have already seen that these hospital personnel are people of faith who bring their own needs to God and petition for His guidance in their work. When we asked them if they "regularly pray" *for* their patients, the priests and Sisters gave a unanimous affirmative answer, but the proportionate affirmative answers decreased to less than seven out of ten for nurses and less than six out of ten for physicians.[9]

Praying for the welfare of a patient implies a relationship with God wherever the praying person happens to be. This may be done anywhere, if not in the hospital chapel, then at least out of the context of the sickroom. A still more personal and spiritual involvement is implied when the hospital personnel pray *with* the sick people. The chaplains, both male and female, report, as expected, that they sometimes pray with the patients they visit.[10] This is true also for nine out of ten of the religious Sisters in nursing. In spite of a few prayerful exceptions among the doctors, we found that physicians are about half as likely (36 percent) as laywomen nurses (76 percent) to report that they sometimes pray with the sick patient.

Spiritual Communication

The infrequency with which physicians pray with their patients bespeaks not only the professional specificity of their medical role but also the general shyness that characterizes the American interpretation of religion. This is reminiscent of Granger Westberg's story of his early attempt to involve the religious concern of a physician with a patient. The doctor replied: "I don't know anything about your business, Reverend. I make it a point to keep off the subject of religion. I can't tell you how to run your affairs." [11] There is evidence that this professional aloofness is breaking down, as suggested in the words of William Reed: "Both the physician and the psychiatrist must see the clergyman in a new light as an ally and not someone simply to be called in for last rites, a prayer, or reassurance prior to death." [12] Despite this apparent reluctance to become involved in the personal prayer patterns of the sick patients, the majority of the medical personnel—more nurses than physicians—say that they feel competent to talk about religion with their patients. This does not mean that they consider themselves accomplished theologians or trained catechists, but it bespeaks a certain confidence that they are familiar with the ordinary "God-talk" that may be called for in the hospital situation. They appear to have a self-image vis-à-vis religious knowledge quite different from that of Westberg's doctor, who was most willing to admit ignorance about God and religion. In both cases, however, it is likely that the physician who "talks religion" feels that he does this on a personal level on a matter that is fully outside the expectations of the professional medical role. From this perspective, it is easy to conclude that religion has nothing to do with healing, and is simply one among many topics of informal personal conversations. Thus a scholarly professor of nursing has remarked that "it is tempting to feel all-powerful and believe that the sole source for healing lies with the healer and the external manipulation of medicine." [13]

Even though these medical professionals think that they

are able to carry on a religious conversation with sick people, they confess in interviews that most of the time they are too busy to do so. In the concrete routine of everyday life in the hospital, they are deeply involved with the immediate needs of the patients. They have to "keep their wits about them," as one conscientious surgeon remarked. Perhaps prayer would take their minds off their work; and one could just as well say that work takes their minds off prayer. Responsible health care requires concentration on the immediate task and the avoidance of any type of distraction. People who say that they pray for God's guidance in their work, as the great majority of these medical professionals say they do, should not have difficulty in combining prayer and work. In the event that a conversation raises complicated religious or theological questions, they can always call on someone from the pastoral-care department.

Most medical personnel, as well as their patients, are not able to articulate their religious concepts in clear, ordinary communication. Perhaps only a minority of hospital patients are comfortable in using traditional "religious language," although they seem able to speak clearly regarding their concerns about the meaning of life and sickness and pain.[14] In the church-related hospital, however, the great majority of the professional personnel may be expected to have some acquaintance with religious vocabularies. In spite of this, secular culture has so privatized religion and its expressions that many Americans are reluctant, if not bashful, to speak of God. It is almost as though the right to privacy denies anyone else the right to raise the subject of God, religion, or prayer. Occasionally, one hears that the more recently trained chaplains who are now moving into hospital pastoral-care teams are almost in fear of "imposing" religion on the sick patients. And as one experienced, but critical, chaplain remarked, "they spend so much time practicing psychology that they never get around to their spiritual task." A social worker spoke of a minister who "believed a clergyman should remain remote, offer religion but never himself," and added that "here religious service consisted exclusively of a nonpersonalized religious ritual." [15] In this instance, the chaplain was aloof not only from the patient but also from the health-care professionals in the hospital.

A psychiatric social worker whom we interviewed was vehemently insistent that there be a closer rapport between the medical personnel and the pastoral personnel. In her concept of health care, she argued particularly that the gap between chaplains and nurses has to be narrowed. "Historically nurses have been healers, and chaplains have been the heralds of Jesus Christ. I think the time has come when nurses need also to be heralds as well as healers, and chaplains have to be healers in addition to heralds." This close relationship between medicine and religion, between spirituality and health care centers around the belief in God as the ultimate Healer. "The question is that whatever their role—social worker, nurse, doctor, pastor—do they believe they have the power in Jesus' name to bring comfort and healing and surcease of pain?" The same holistic and religious concept is stressed by William Reed: "The Ministry of Healing should never be conducted apart from the doctor and the nurse who, along with an enlightened clergy, should be the agencies of the healing love of Jesus Christ." [16]

Practically all of the health-care professionals in these church-related hospitals are believers in the existence and providence of God, but strength and intensity of this religious belief varies from person to person. We have seen that in general they have some faith in the power of prayer; most of them pray for God's guidance in their daily work, and they pray for their patients. We asked them the blunt question whether they think that "prayer is a helpful part of the healing process for people in pain." None of the respondents disagreed with this statement, but the percentage of those who "strongly agree" is twice as high among the religious Sisters (61 percent) as it is among the physicians (29 percent). The interpretation of this concept may be subjective regarding the patient's own response to the healing quality of prayer, or it may be objective regarding the intervention of God in the healing process of the patient.

Healing from God

Traditionally, prayer is recognized as an appeal for God's assistance to meet the needs of human creatures. The prayer of petition is probably recited more frequently than any other type. If these health-care professionals believe that God answers prayers during the process of alleviating pain, they are likely also to believe that ultimately, in some indefinite fashion, God is responsible for all healing. We asked them then if they believe that "in the long run, all healing is attributable to the providence of God." This did not get a universal affirmative, even from the professional religious. Three-quarters of the chaplains and Sisters agreed with this statement, as compared to three out of five (61 percent) of the physicians, nurses, and social workers. It is certainly understandable that the latter group would want to reserve some of the curative achievement for themselves. Medical professionals are well aware that they and their colleagues have worked diligently—and with some success—in alleviating the discomfort of patients. In fact, the focus of their training and experience has been precisely the healing of sick people, and they probably feel that some of the "credit" for healing should go to the health professionals, even when they know that ultimately all people and their problems are in the hands of God.

Does the spiritual dimension of health care actually have an effect on sick people? Are the consolations of religion in some way measurable in the hospital setting? One of the most dramatic examples of the power of prayer and the consolations of religion occurs regularly in many religious hospitals in the morning hours before surgery. A survey of patients in a Rochester hospital several years ago revealed that "a visit from the chaplain before surgery ranked high on most patients' lists irrespective of their denominations." [17] One hospital chaplain reported that most surgeons are appreciative of this preoperative contact that the minister has with the patient. "Several of the doctors told me that they have to use less than half of the usual anesthetic for patients who have been prayed with because they are so relaxed." A certain amount of fear and tension is normal especially after the surgeon, accompanied by an intern, has just described to the patient what the operation will entail. The presence and prayers of the clergyperson provide an assurance that is of great help to the patients.[18]

In researching the incidence of healing attributable directly to prayer and to God, we asked whether faith healers and Pentecostals were permitted to visit patients in these hospitals. Such visits were allowed in most of the hospitals under two conditions: first, that the patient had requested it and secondly, that the prayer ceremony be conducted quietly and without disturbance to other patients. In several instances, students from nearby Bible colleges applied to do volunteer work for the hospital but attempted to "convert sinners to the Lord." One hospital chaplain, himself a Baptist minister, said that when he first arrived, "groups of them were going from room to room, visiting, shouting, preaching, healing, and it was my responsibility to put a stop to this. Of course, they accused me of being in league with Satan." The organized healing ministry, of which Oral Roberts is probably the most famous exemplar, has reached more sophisticated levels among the mainline Protestant churches.[19] It has also, as we noted earlier, become hesitantly popular among Roman Catholics, whose foremost spokesman for prayer healing is Francis MacNutt.

In the survey of church-related hospital personnel, we asked "have you ever seen a case of 'miraculous' remission (that is, one that was unexpected or unexplained by doctors)?" The majority (62 percent) said they were not aware of anything like this happening in their experience. A small minority (12 percent) who said that such remissions had occurred did not provide a description of the event. We were interested only in the remaining one-fourth (26 percent) who had witnessed such a "cure" and provided a description of it.[20] Proportionately more nurses (32 percent) reported such occurrences, and it is an interesting fact that the same proportion of physicians (19.6 percent) as of chaplains (20.6 percent) said they had seen this kind of unexpected cure. One nurse told of a "small infant with a congenital heart problem complicated by pneumonia. The doctor gave up on her recovery, but she lived and is now about thirteen years of age. Just recently she survived her second open heart surgery." A chaplain told of the patient who had "diagnosis of carcinoma of the gall bladder. The surgeon who did the operation gave the patient no more than three months to live. The surgery was done one year ago and the remission holds complete. The doctor has no explanation and himself marvels." A physician tells of a young girl who "was about to enter the convent and was found to have a malignant lesion of the trachea, which was inoperable. As a last resort she was given radiation, and has been in remission now for over ten years. This is the closest to a miracle I have seen. She is a nun now in New Mexico."

There is a difference between acceptance of the fact that "medical science does not have all the answers," and the forthright statement that whatever the physicians cannot explain in the recovery of the sick person must be the direct intervention of God. There is a difference also between the unexplained cure that happens as a consequence of fervent prayer, and the cure that "just happens." A pastoral associate told us of a religious Sister in her order who was in stage four of Hodgkin's disease. "That's the final and fatal stage. A charismatic lady came to the hospital, laid hands on her, prayed with her and said she would be healed. Now she is back down here at the hospital for all kinds of tests. They can't find anything wrong with her. There is no evidence of Hodgkin's disease." A certain skepticism is current among Americans, even regular churchgoers, about the intervention of God in the healing process. The skepticism tends to lessen among health professionals after they see "unexpected" improvements in sick patients. Doctors who have encountered medically inexplicable healings, says

Emily Neal, used to attribute this to faulty diagnosis. "To-day many of these same men, now familiar with the healing phenomenon, believe that the continued affirmation that the medically-diagnosed disease never existed in the first place constitutes an unwarranted indictment against modern diagnostic methods and medical skill, and is neither an honest nor a realistic approach to the subject." [21]

Notes

1 Dennis Saylor, *And You Visited Me* (Medford: Morse Press, 1979), p. 196.

2 Joseph M. Dolan, *Give Comfort to My People* (New York: Paulist Press, 1977), p. 11.

3 Harley S. Smyth, "In Word and Deed: The Witness of the Catholic Hospital," *Catholic Hospital* 6 (January-February 1978): 12–13.

4 See Gerald Niklas and Charlotte Stefanics, *Ministry to the Hospitalized* (New York: Paulist Press, 1975), chap. 2, "Ministering to the Sick through Prayer."

5 For a broader perspective, see Barbara Thomas, "Corporate Evangelization: Pooling Generosity and Competence," *Hospital Progress* 59 (August 1978): 67–68, 73.

6 Heije Faber, *Pastoral Care in the Modern Hospital* (Philadelphia: Westminster, 1977), "Faith and Illness," pp. 38–47.

7 A different image was portrayed by the personnel director of one hospital who feared that a union was being formed and who said "the nurses are coached to be selfish and dissatisfied even before they come to work here."

8 Arthur Henley, "Ministers and Medicine," *Physician's World* 2, no. 2 (February 1974): 48–52.

9 See J. T. Hall, "A Dynamic Concept of Prayer for the Sick," *Pastoral Psychology* 20, no. 197 (October 1969): 45.

10 Raymond G. Carey, *Hospital Chaplains: Who Needs Them?* (St. Louis: Catholic Hospital Association, 1972), found that only 8 percent of chaplains put a "high value" on praying for and with patients. Significantly, physicians, nurses, and patients themselves were about four times more likely than the clergy to give this high evaluation.

11 Granger E. Westberg, *Minister and Doctor Meet* (New York: Harper and Row, 1961), p. 3.

12 William S. Reed, *Surgery of the Soul* (Old Tappan: Revell, 1969), p. 109.

13 Florence M. Schubert, "The Function of Religion in Medical Care," in *Medicine and Religion: Strategies of Care,* ed. Donald W. Shriver (Pittsburgh: University of Pittsburgh Press, 1980), pp. 105–11.

14 See Harmon L. Smith, "The Minister as Consultant to the Medical Team," *Journal of Religion and Health* 14, no. 1 (January 1975).

15 Marion Kahn, "Some Observations on the Role of Religion in Illness," *Social Work* 3 (July 1958): 83–89. Paul Pruyser remarks that "pastors are sometimes wary about the God-talk of their clients, going out of their way to avoid it themselves." *The Minister as Diagnostician* (Philadelphia: Westminster, 1976), p. 91.

16 William Reed, *Surgery of the Soul* (Old Tappan: Revell, 1969), p. 56.

17 Cashel Weiler, "Patients Evaluate Pastoral Care," *Hospital Progress* 56 (April 1975): 34–35, 38.

18 See James S. Miller, "Therapies Ministers Use," *The Christian Century* 94 (25 May 1977).

19 A popular and reliable study is David E. Harrell, *All Things Are Possible: The Healing and Charismatic Revivals in Modern America* (Bloomington: Indiana University Press, 1975), p. 5, who writes that "the charismatic movement became a vital but amorphous phenomenon, ranging from tent healers and old-time pentecostals to sophisticated Episcopalians and Roman Catholics who discovered anew the gifts of the Holy Spirit."

20 Healing of physical infirmities had been witnessed in 37 percent of the charismatic prayer groups we studied in *The Catholic Cult of the Paraclete* (New York: Sheed and Ward, 1975), pp. 127–32.

21 Emily Gardiner Neal, *God Can Heal You Now* (Englewood Cliffs: Prentice-Hall, 1958), p. 120.

Chapter 7
Sisters and Nurses

The occupational role of women has been changing rapidly in the recent past of American society.[1] Women are given assurances by affirmative-action employers that they will have job opportunities equal to those of males in the work force. Nevertheless, there is still the stereotype and the actuality of certain kinds of "women's work" as exemplified in some areas of the helping professions: social work, teaching, and nursing. Even in these occupations, both in the churches and in the larger society, the managerial positions are still largely in the hands of males. The statement of Vatican II that "women claim for themselves an equity with men before the law and in fact," is still short of achievement.[2]

Our specific quest for the spiritual dimensions of health care focuses here on the women who are engaged in the personal service to the sick in church-related hospitals.[3] Among Catholics many religious women hold responsible positions of administration in the hospital system, just as they do in the field of education, and it is both because of the large numbers of women in hospital work, and because of the large size of the Catholic hospital system that in this chapter the discussion will center largely on the Sisters and nurses in Catholic health-care facilities. If spirituality is exemplified anywhere in the Catholic hospital system it ought to be found among the women who have dedicated their lives to God in the service of sick and needy people. Historically, there gradually developed groups of Christian women who formed religious communities specifically dedicated to care of the sick and needy. In later years, they

96

have been joined by more and more dedicated and trained laywomen in the nursing ministry to people in pain.

The Helping Professions

Vocational opportunities for women within the American Catholic Church have been in the traditional female occupational roles, with the largest number in the parochial school system. A survey of female religious personnel, made about two decades ago, showed that 81 percent were teaching, 12 percent were in hospital work, and the rest in several forms of social work.[4] About nine out of ten of all full-time teachers in the Catholic school system were female (61 percent Sisters and 28 percent laywomen). Teaching is still the Catholic occupation that employs the largest number of women, but the proportion of laywomen teachers has increased significantly, while the number of elementary parochial schools has declined. Women continue to outnumber men in the church's institutions of education and social service, but numerous factors account for the shift of emphasis indicated in the following table. We have already seen that the numbers of Catholic hospitals and schools of nursing have dramatically declined. With the lower birthrate, there has been less need for the maintenance of orphanages and infant asylums. On the other hand, the growing proportion of the elderly has resulted in the establishment of more convalescent and nursing homes for the aged.

TABLE 1

Distribution of establishments in which Catholic women religious were employed, 1963 and 1980

	1963	1980
Parochial elementary schools	10,322	7,847
Hospitals and sanatoria	946	720
Schools of nursing	342	121
Homes for the aged	357	497
Orphanages and infant asylums	258	207
Protective institutions	134	127

Every large diocese in the country has a variety of institutions to carry on the corporal works of mercy, to promote both evangelization and social justice. They employ professional social workers, most of whom are women. These organizations carry different labels while covering approximately the same kind of services to the needs of the people. Most of them had originally been under the title of Catholic Charities but are also known as the department of Christian Service, Family Life Bureau, Program for Refugees and Migrants, and often there are special committees for types of handicapped persons, the lame, the blind, and the deaf. None of these apostolic ministries could continue to function successfully if there were not large numbers of conscientious and trained women available.[5] When these diocesan bureaus and committees first began, they were almost always headed by a clergyman—a monsignor if the post was prestigious enough—and may have included one or two professionally trained religious Sisters. As the needs became more pressing and these institutions increased in size, they employed more and more laywomen social workers. As the helping professions demanded further training and more extensive education, the criteria for employment began to place almost as much emphasis on the woman's professional competence as on the fact that she was of the Catholic faith.

The feminist movement has brought forth many legitimate complaints about discriminatory sexism in organized religion, and particularly in the Roman Catholic Church.[6] There is, however, one positive aspect that is frequently overlooked. It is only within the Catholic Church that large numbers of women, religious Sisters, hold important positions in the faculty and administration of women's colleges. This is true also of the other establishments listed in the above table, where nuns held responsibility for hospitals, orphanages, old folks' homes, and other facilities in Catholic charities. Before the Second Vatican Council, there was occupational upward mobility for Catholic women, but it was almost exclusively for the members of religious congregations.[7] Since the council, and especially since the ordination of women to the Episcopalian priesthood and the concomitant decline of male priestly vocations, the apostolic ministry of women has increased enormously. The proportion of female seminarians among theology students is providing a steady stream of aspirants for parochial, diocesan, and institutional positions previously held exclusively by males.

While the sex distribution of the respondents to this study is not meant to reflect the actual proportions of men and women in these hospitals, we find that almost two-thirds of them (64 percent) are female. The listing of hospitals in the *Catholic Directory* usually provides the names of the administrator and the priest chaplain, and the number of religious Sisters and nurses. It does not reveal how many males are employed at the hospital, but simple observation and experience in these hospitals demonstrate that females far outnumber males.[8] Relatively few men are entering the nursing profession, but the number of women physicians is gradually increasing, since the medical schools have come into compliance with equal-opportunity legislation.[9] There continues to be a predominance of males, however, on the medical staff of all general hospitals, whether public, proprietary, or church-related.

Fewer Women Religious

When Cardinal Suenens published his popular book, *Nun in the World,* in 1963,[10] the American women religious were busy about improved professional training and an expanded apostolate. Various options were earnestly discussed, and we were reminded that "the hospital apostolate is almost unlimited: contact with patients in apostolic follow-up in their homes; contact with the families of patients, often themselves spiritual patients for our ministrations; home visiting of the sick and aged in the parish; organizing retreats and recollection days for different categories of patients, for doctors, nurses, personnel; organizing action groups of the same categories for training in the apostolate and in their roles in the church." [11] It can be said that the enthusiasm for *aggiornamento* had prevailed among these American women well before John XXIII came on the world scene to popularize the term.

It was a time of great aspirations, when almost unlimited opportunities for development lay before the American congregations of women religious. In 1966, the year after the close of the Second Vatican Council, the number of religious Sisters reached its all-time peak, 181,421. By 1980 this number had shrunk to 126,517, and the repercussions of this shrinkage were felt in all the church apostolates where the nuns had been making their greatest occupational contribution. Fewer young women were entering the novitiates of religious congregations to replace those who had died and especially to fill the roles of the large numbers who had resigned from the sisterhoods.[12] There is no need to discuss here the reasons for this decline in the numbers of vocations among women religious, a decline which is apparent also among all Catholic male church professionals: priests, Brothers, seminarians. Meanwhile, the American Catholic population continued to expand: new dioceses were established and new parishes were opened. Because of the shortage of Sisters to staff the elementary and secondary schools many of them had to close down and others had to employ a growing echelon of lay teachers. The lack of religious women to staff and administer Catholic schools of nursing was one of the reasons why so many of them went out of existence. Many changes of personnel occurred also in the Catholic hospital system.

With the exception of three institutions operated by congregations of religious Brothers, all of the church-related hospitals from which we obtained completed questionnaires are under the auspices of religious congregations of women. Some of the largest of these hospitals have more than twenty-five nuns on the staff,[13] but the average number for all of them is 11.1 women religious. In other words, the 297 Sisters' hospitals of this survey have 3,300 women religious ministering to the patients in various capacities. The

TABLE 2
Occupational distribution of 3,300 religious
Sisters in 297 Catholic hospitals

	Number	Percent
Bedside nurses	556	16.9
Pastoral care	657	19.9
Supervisors	905	27.4
Other positions	1,182	35.8

above table reveals their proportional distribution in the
several categories of hospital work.

Most of the religious Sisters who took hospital training and
became registered nurses say that they had originally intended to exercise their apostolic ministry as bedside nurses.
Indeed, when the oldest of these hospitals was first established, practically all of the bedside nursing was done by
religious Sisters. This was the direction in which their vocation lay, but circumstances decreed otherwise. Over the
decades, as the hospitals expanded and the number of patients multiplied, many laywomen were trained in nursing,
while many of the Sisters became head nurses and supervisors or moved into administrative positions. At the present
time, and among the church-related hospitals answering this
survey, almost three out of ten (28 percent) have no Sisters at
all in the role of bedside nursing. A young laywoman nurse
in a Catholic hospital of over 350 beds told us that she knew
of only three bedside nursing Sisters out of the 238 nurses in
the hospital. She felt that the Sisters have certain educational
and professional advantages in belonging to religious congregations. "They don't have to pay for their own training
and education, and they are able to get bachelor's and master's degrees in nursing. They get to be supervisors on the
different floors and wards of the hospital. The Sisters, of
course, are the administrators of the hospital." It is true that
the Sister nurses answering our questionnaires are more
than twice as likely (89 percent) as the laywomen nurses (43
percent) to have attained an academic degree.

Many of the hospitals conducted by religious congregations of women continue to have a Sister as president, chief executive, or administrator, but there is a gradually increasing proportion that now employ trained lay persons in positions of top management.[14] From the point of view of personal and spiritual contact with sick people, however, the most significant switch for Sisters has been away from the immediate bedside care of the sick. It is interesting that the largest single category of sisters in Table 2 is made up of women in "other" positions, which constitute an interminable listing in the finance office, the cafeteria, the laundry, the laboratory, and elsewhere in the hospital.[15] This does not mean that all of these positions are filled by Sisters who were formerly involved in nursing. As a matter of fact, most of them were trained and educated for nonmedical occupations.

Non-Sister Nurses

As the numbers of women religious decline, and as they move from bedside nursing to supervisory positions and to other hospital functions, their prayerful influence on the patients will be funneled through the nurses working under their direction. Whether or not this will lessen the influence of the consolations of religion to sick people will probably depend on the extent to which the laywomen nurses fulfill the spiritual functions of the Catholic hospital system. "If a Catholic health facility is to witness to Christian values today, it must do so through the services rendered and values expressed by its employees in their contacts with patients and fellow staff." [16] There is no reason to expect that the proportion of Catholics, whether on the medical staff or in other employment, will decrease. Hospitals will become more and more a ministry of the laity, and these are the people who must be the chief witnesses to Christian values.

At the present time in these Catholic hospitals, the vast majority of the nurses are laywomen, and almost one-third of them (32 percent) are not members of the Catholic Church. For the most part, however, they are Christian believers and have affiliation with various Protestant churches. The comparisons we make here between the Sisters and non-Sisters who are nurses do not revolve around their technical and medical skills. The non-Sisters are on the average two years younger than the Sisters, have been in hospital work for fewer years, and fewer have academic degrees in nursing. We assume, however, that all these nurses have been tested for professional competence and are retained in employment on the basis of experience and proven ability to deal with sick people. The comparative analysis then centers on questions of faith, spirituality, the consolations of religion. One of the puzzling differences between these two categories of nurses is that the laywomen seem to have a higher appreciation of the hospital's effort to bring religion to patients. When we asked them "in general, how is spiritual ministry to the sick rated in this hospital?" the lay nurses were much more likely (70 percent) than the Sister nurses (54 percent) to give a high rating. We asked them also to make a general assessment of pastoral care at their hospital,[17] and again the non-Sisters were more likely (56 percent to 31 percent) than the Sisters to say that it is "excellent." Indeed, one-fifth of the Sisters assessed it as "only fair."

The statistical comparison showing that the religious women give pastoral care and spiritual ministry a relatively low rating is at first glance an unexpected finding and requires some explanation. One may speculate that because of their deep religious training and their professed spiritual ideals the Sisters entertain loftier expectations of the hospital's spiritual ministry and place greater demands on the people in the pastoral-care department. In other words, they are less easily satisfied with the quality of spiritual care than are the non-Sisters. It is likely also that they pay closer attention and know more about the actual ministry that is being conducted for the religious benefit of the sick patients. Religious practices are more central to their whole way of life, both personal and professional, and this seems certain to sharpen their awareness of others.

The proportional responses were switched when we asked the much more personal question about their own spirituality. When we asked to what extent these hospital nurses considered spiritual ministry to the sick an aspect of their own daily work, a higher percentage of Sisters (87 percent) than of non-Sisters (71 percent) said that they consider it "essential." There was practically the same proportional difference (87 percent to 73 percent) of agreement to the statement that "you can't be a good health professional unless you have a spiritual perspective on life." We proposed also the statement that "the holistic approach in modern health care has to include spiritual ministration to patients." Here again the Sisters were much more likely (80 percent) than the non-Sisters (57 percent) to say that they "strongly agree" with this statement.

The holistic approach to healing is intimately related to the spiritual ministry of health care, and both concepts—holistic and spiritual—help to sustain an environment of love and concern in the hospital.[18] All departments of the institution are contributory to the therapeutic community, but the role of nursing appears to be qualitatively more demanding for the benefit of the sick person. It is clear that the religious conceptualization of the health-care profession is of greater significance to the women religious than it is to the non-Sisters. Nevertheless, many of the laywomen nurses give the impression of deep spiritual solicitude. A clinical nurse specialist who has been friend and counselor of many young nurses said of them: "There is a manner about them; they are comfortable with themselves and this is reflected in the way they are with peers, with patients, and with families. I mean there is a love there that is radiated to others."

Both types of nurses report that they pray for God's guidance in the work they do daily with sick people, and this tends to be a relatively brief petition for divine help rather than a formal meditative prayer. Practically all of the Sisters, and about seven out of ten of the non-Sisters report that they "regularly pray" for their patients, asking God to relieve their pain and anxieties. In approximately the same comparative proportions they also say that they "sometimes pray" with the patients. Aside from the pastoral-care department, which now also includes women, the hospital nurses constitute the main instrument for bringing the consolations of religion to people in pain. In the church-related hospitals this ministry is carried more and more by laywomen.

Notes

1 This chapter is a revision of an article of the same title, "Sisters and Nurses," *Review for Religious* 38, no. 6 (November 1979): 839–45.

2 *Gaudium et Spes* (7 December 1965), ART. 9. The first papal statement on equal rights of women came from John XXIII in *Pacem in Terris* (10 April 1963), ART. 41.

3 In European hospitals, all nurses are called "Sister," whether they are deaconesses, nuns, or laywomen. The Dutch Protestant Pastor Heije Faber uses this term but sometimes distinguishes between Protestant minister and Catholic priest in the hospital setting. See *Pastoral Care in the Modern Hospital* (Philadelphia: Westminster, 1977).

4 See Joseph H. Fichter, *Religion as an Occupation* (Notre Dame: University of Notre Dame Press, 1961), pp. 145–48.

5 The demand for equal opportunity and apostolic recognition is most vocal in the movement for ordination. See A. M. Gardiner, ed., *Women and Catholic Priesthood: An Expanded Vision* (New York: Paulist Press, 1976); also Fran Ferder, *Called to Break Bread?* (Mt. Rainier: Quixote Center, 1978).

6 See Mary Daly, *The Church and the Second Sex* (New York: Harper and Row, 1968), chap. 1, "The Case Against the Church."

7 See Sally Cunneen, *Sex: Female; Religion: Catholic* (New York: Holt, Rinehart & Winston, 1968), chap. 7, "Nuns in Evolution."

8 In 1978, females constituted 92.9 percent of registered nurses, dietitians, and therapists. *Statistical Abstract of U.S. Bureau of the Census.*

9 In 1977, women made up only 9.8 percent of American physi-

cians, but in 1980 the American Association of Medical Colleges reported that entering freshmen, the first-year class of 1984, contained 28.9 percent women. See *The New Physician* 30, no. 1 (January 1981): 18.

10 Leon-Josef Cardinal Suenens, *Nun in the World* (Philadelphia: Westminster, 1963).

11 Gertrude Donnelly, *The Sister Apostle* (Notre Dame: Fides, 1964), p. 21.

12 For a sociological analysis of this phenomenon, see Helen Ebaugh, *Out of the Cloister* (Austin: University of Texas Press, 1977). For an earlier study of "defections," see Joseph H. Fichter, *Religion As an Occupation* (Notre Dame: University of Notre Dame Press, 1961), chap. 8, "Giving Up the Vocation."

13 For the correct definition of Sisters and nuns, see *New Catholic Encylopedia*, vol. 10, W. B. Ryan, "Nun," p. 575, and vol. 13, "Sister," p. 261.

14 Problems of reorganization and retrenchment in the church-related hospital systems continue to be under research scrutiny. See, for example, Vincent DiPaolo, "Catholic Congregations Contemplate Forming a Regional Hospital Network," *Modern Healthcare* 8 (August 1978): 8–9; also M. Concilia Moran, "Sponsorship: The Uneasy Question," *Hospital Progress* 59 (October 1978): 52–55, 70.

15 The variety of people who deal directly or indirectly with the hospital patients is listed by Beverly Du Gas, *Introduction to Patient Care* (Philadelphia: Saunders, 1977), p. 104.

16 William Kenney and Charles Ceronsky, "Developing Christian Values in a Catholic Health Facility," *Hospital Progress* 55 (October 1974): 32, 36–37.

17 A similar question asked of patients in a large Catholic hospital in Minnesota elicited responses that differed according to the church affiliation of the patients. See Cashel Weiler, "Patients Evaluate Pastoral Care," *Hospital Progress* 56 (April 1975): 34–35, 38.

18 A description of such a hospital community is given by Jeanette Verzillo, "A Program for Caring," *Supervisor Nurse* (July 1980): 10–16. An important goal of Catholic health facilities is "forming community" as a network of support and solidarity, according to Kevin O'Rourke, "Developing a Strong Catholic Identity," *Hospital Progress* 57 (July 1976): 88–90.

Chapter 8

Pastoral Care

The chaplains, both male and female, in the pastoral-care departments, are at the heart of the organized Christian enterprise to bring the consolations of religion to suffering hospital patients. The concept of the "healing community," in which everybody brings a spiritual dimension to each task and to each patient, does not replace the designated chaplain.[1] The clergy represent Christ, religion, and the church in a special and symbolic way which continues to be recognized by the sick laity. Even the smallest church-related hospital has an assigned chaplain, sometimes a local priest, rabbi, or minister who is on call or may also visit the sick at regular hours.

Three-quarters of the hospitals reporting in this survey had organized pastoral-care departments, and they average 4.5 pastoral ministers, or associates, in each department. This seems remarkable progress since 1971, when the Catholic Hospital Association surveyed the American chaplaincies and found that only one-fifth (21 percent) then had departments of pastoral care.[2] At that time in the Catholic hospitals, only ordained priests were counted as members of the department; at the present time, we find numerous "pastoral associates," most of whom are religious Sisters, and some are laywomen.[3] Even now, however, the person who is officially designated the chaplain may not be a woman.

The New Breed

The typical "job description" for the Catholic hospital chaplains continues to say that he is an ordained priest who "provides daily for the administration of the sacraments: baptism, penance, eucharist, and the Annointing of the Sick. He is available on any appropriate occasion to celebrate Mass for patients and personnel." [4] The code had "directives of a religious nature which concern the reception and administration of the sacraments and the reverent disposal of amputated members and immature babies." [5] Only an ordained person could perform the traditional sacramental and ritual role. In many Catholic health facilities, it had been performed faithfully by hospital chaplains who had no special training for this work. Often they acted as spiritual director for the religious community of Sisters operating the hospital and were appointed because they themselves needed medical attention, or had been found inadequate to fulfill other roles of the ordained ministry in parishes, schools, and missions.

The modern average clergyman engaged in hospital pastoral care is younger than the traditional chaplain and has also had some form of Clinical Pastoral Education. Among the clergy chaplain respondents to this study, the majority (71 percent) have been in hospital work for less than ten years, and they seem to have shifted positions fairly recently. Half of them (51 percent) moved into the position at their present hospital in the past three years. This seems to reflect the stated caution that there is " a need for clinical experience for those working in the field of pastoral care and counselling. The idea that a person could be an adequate minister if he 'read theology' and learned the appropriate rituals gradually gave way to a recognition that adequate pastoral care involved knowledge and understanding of a wider spectrum of human experience." [6]

Although there are still some traditionalists who insist that "prayer and the sacraments are enough," the great majority of people in the hospital ministry favor professional training. Nevertheless, controversy revolves around the nature of the training in clinical pastoral education. Interviews with hospital chaplains who have gone through one or more units of such education have revealed divergent estimates of this training experience. Some of them have complained that there was no "faith content" in the courses they took, that God, religion, and spirituality were totally excluded from this training and that the emphasis was on the process of counseling. One clergyman reported that he had not been accepted into the training course until he promised not to mention God, nor to touch any patient, during the training period. One Sister was told that she should not wear her religious habit, or any outward symbol like a cross or medal, while in the Clinical Pastoral Education course.

The fact that the movement for clinical pastoral training was of Protestant origin and started in mental hospitals by Congregational clergyman Anton Boisen, may be the reason why some Catholic chaplains were reluctant to accept it.[7] Even in the late sixties at one large Catholic hospital there were problems among the chaplains. "The polarization of department members revealed little foundation for cooperation and organization. The Protestant chaplains doubted the Catholic chaplains' competence because they were not CPE certified, while the Catholic chaplains believed that the CPE certified Protestant chaplains were too entrenched in a psychologically rather than spiritually oriented ministry."[8] It would be a mistake to think of this as a typical confrontation between Catholic and Protestant hospital chaplains. Indeed, a Protestant author, Don Browning, complained that the educational programs for pastoral-care directors were "becoming more and more preoccupied with issues relating to counselling techniques and less and less interested as professionals in issues relating to ethics, theology and the philosophy of religion."[9]

The need for professional specialization was recognized as much by Catholic chaplains as by Protestant chaplains, and there developed a parallel system of training and certification by the Office of Chaplain Services of the United States Catholic Conference. Nevertheless, there continued to be some dissatisfaction with the emphasis on counseling techniques and procedures, and with the lack of attention to faith and theology. The students in training report that peculiar warnings are issued to them in the clinical pastoral course that they must not "impose" religion on sick people. The chaplain must meet the patient, as they say, "where the patient is." He must wait cautiously until the patient is "ready" to talk about God and prayer and religion. As we noted earlier, there is little spiritual consolation in an approach that is based on the assumption that any secular topic of conversation is much more interesting and attractive to the sick person than religion—and in our contemporary urban secular culture this may well be true. From this perspective, the chaplain is not seen as the pastor sent by God with a mission to evangelize, or to bring the "good news" of salvation to suffering people. Paul Pruyser has made this point as clearly as any other expert. He complains that at pastoral-care conferences the pastors tend to use psychological language, repeating "stultified" words like depression, paranoid, hysterical. "When clients clearly sought pastoral answers to questions of conscience or correct belief, the pastors tended either to ignore these questions or to translate them quickly into psychological or social interactional subtleties." [10]

Psychologist Bernard Spilka and his associates find that there is a trend toward secularism among the clergy, a rejection of traditional spiritual roles and a preference for the role of comforter and counselor. Their research shows the ministers often neglecting whatever competence they had in religious knowledge or in pastoral theology and simply imitating the language and concepts of clinical psychology. One of the unexpected results of this situation is that some priests and ministers do not know "what to say" when they are confronted with people in pain. They are ill at ease with sick people, especially with the dying.[11] They exchange a few quick pleasantries and leave as soon as possible. This type of person is sometimes the parish clergyman who "drops by" to visit one of the sick parishioners either at home or in the hospital, or in the Catholic hospital it may be the busy old-time hospital chaplain who simply says a quick prayer in Latin while giving the patient holy communion.

Sisters and Laity

Until recently the chaplain role in both church-related and nonsectarian hospitals has seldom been filled by women, even by those who are ordained ministers, although women—much more so than men—were regular visitors to the sick. One of the most interesting changes that has occurred in Catholic hospital personnel is the attraction of religious Sisters and Brothers to the role of pastoral care. Robert Wheelock remarks that the Sister as pastoral associate is "rapidly becoming one of the most vital and indispensable persons in our Catholic hospital." [12] In the hospitals here under study we note that there are more Sisters in pastoral care (657) than in bedside nursing (556). What is probably more surprising is that religious women outnumber clergymen (447) among the 1,104 persons engaged in pastoral care in these hospitals.

The women religious in hospital pastoral care tend to be older than the ministers and have had many more years of experience in the field of health care. When we asked them how long they had been in this kind of work we found that the Sister chaplains are six times more likely (42 percent to 7 percent) to say that they have been in the hospital apostolate for more than twenty years. Many of them shifted into pastoral care as they approached the age of retirement from active nursing duty. There are exceptions, of course, like the very popular Sister who said she had been a high-school teacher, treasurer of her province, and administrative secretary of the hospital before she moved into her current role as pastoral associate.

David McPhee has described that earlier period when Catholic hospitals had "Sister-visitors," who were usually elderly religious in semiretirement. "Many were former teachers or nurses and, while not specifically trained in pastoral care, they were able to provide friendly support on their daily rounds to patient areas." [13] These devoted and spiritually wise women continue to bring the consolations of religion to sick patients, and they are especially popular with older Catholics, who disapprove of all the changes going on in the church, like the modernization of nuns' religious habits, and are comfortable with "Sisters who look like Sisters." There were Sister-visitors in the hospitals of this study which did not have a pastoral-care department, as well as in those hospitals to which only one ordained chaplain was assigned. In the present study, we did not include Sister-visitors as members of the formally organized departments of pastoral care. In many instances, their status is not fully defined within the organizational structure of the hospital and they tend to occupy a peripheral, but often highly appreciated, position. Occasionally, a seminarian or religious Brother also performs this function, and more frequently as the lay apostolate and the charismatic movement develop there are specially trained lay volunteers from the local congregations and parishes.[14]

Women religious who are fully accredited as associates in the pastoral-care departments of Catholic hospitals say that in some cases ordained clergymen are reluctant to grant full chaplain status to women. They point out, however, that the old-time Sister-visitors are acceptable to the clergy "because they keep their place." The clergy chaplains who feel threatened are usually those with little formal training, who retain the exclusively ritual and sacramental concept of hospital chaplaincy. A Sister who is an interdenominational chaplain in a large public hospital, and also a supervisor in the CPE training program, spoke disparagingly of some priests who "come in at nine-thirty and go home at three and think they have done a day's work. They have no concept of professional pastoral care."

Experienced women religious point out that the title "chaplain" in Catholic hospitals is reserved for ordained males, while religious Sisters—no matter how well trained and certified—are designated "pastoral associates." From a functional point of view, this designation does not interfere with the actual performance of the pastoral role, except that the unordained woman may not provide sacramental absolution. From a status perspective, it is also true that many older patients, both Protestant and Catholic, have not become accustomed to the spiritual ministry of a "clergywoman." The first qualification to be a Catholic chaplain, as established by the National Association of Catholic Chaplains, is "ordination to the priesthood and continuing ecclesiastical endorsement by the Ordinary of the Diocese or one's religious superior." [15] Until the sacerdotal ordination of women is introduced by the Catholic Church, this primary qualification clearly excludes religious Sisters, or any other women, from becoming full-fledged hospital chaplains. Several Sisters cited the carefully worded "help wanted" adds in the *National Catholic Reporter* that distinguish between the full chaplain and the pastoral associate.

It is an interesting fact that the Protestant-dominated CPE was quicker to accept women trainees, and has educated more Sisters, than the Office of Chaplain Services of the United States Catholic Conference. Both of these are accrediting agencies for training centers and provide certification for individuals who successfully complete the program. It is clear that the professional training provided here and elsewhere does not require ordination. As McPhee states, "priest-chaplains are specialists, not because of their sacramental power, but because of their training in crisis counseling and pastoral therapy." [16] Sacramental ministry is still required and is important, but aside from that, "clinically trained sisters could serve as chaplains with equal competence and responsibility." From this professional perspective, then, women religious are no longer seen as "subservient" to priests in the hospital chaplaincy.

The so-called rivalry that has sometimes been noted between the respective alumni and alumnae of CPE and NACC seems to be gradually abating. The relative emphasis on the psychological rather than the theological—or vice versa—depends upon the particular supervisor of the clinical training program. What makes the "new" pastoral care distinctive seems to be the *process* of relating to the patient rather than the *content* of religion and faith—which is probably assumed to have found nothing "new." It is worth noting that in both instances the training takes place more often in hospitals than in seminaries or universities, and thus reflects a greater medical than theological orientation.[17] Raymond Smith feels it is "mandatory" that it take place in residential training centers where the student has daily "experience of group process and verbatim reporting of patient and staff encounters." [18]

Relations with Medical Staff

A frequent observation by the pastoral-care people we interviewed is that hospitals are now largely dominated by medical men who think of nurses, social workers, Sisters, and clergy as their subordinates. Ivan Illich's comment is more trenchant: "The radical monopoly over health care that the contemporary physician claims now forces him to reassume priestly and royal functions that his ancestors gave up when they became specialized as technical healers." [19] In some instances, it is as though the physicians and surgeons who were once permitted to work in the hospitals are now permitting the religious Sisters and chaplains to work there. Harmon Smith remarks that "the practice of medicine, particularly in the medical center, is widely thought by physicians themselves to be a 'closed shop'; what is sometimes called the 'white-coat mystique' serves, on hospital turf, to remind everyone (including the clergymen) of a hierarchy of functional importance." [20]

From the perspective of the sick patient, the physician takes on large importance because there is no other person or place to turn for relief from pain. People depend on the doctor who begins to act as though he really possesses the authority, confidence, and power that were once attributed to prophets and saints. Smith suggests further that the ministers of religion sometimes view these medical men as "usurpers of a position and prominence and expertise that used to be theirs." The doctors have become the "vested clergy of a new religion," while the pastors and chaplains tend to be deferential toward this new priesthood. There is no question that the status of physicians and surgeons has been greatly inflated in modern times and that many people accord them almost reverential prestige. Arnold Hutschnecker remarks that "in other people's minds the doctor has inherited the mantle of the high priest, and some physicians are not averse to trying it on now and then." [21]

In this study of church-related hospitals, we asked all the respondents whether "the ministers of religion get full cooperation here from physicians and surgeons." A majority of the chaplains—more male (68 percent) than female (56 percent)—answered in the affirmative. When we sought the answer from another point of view and asked the respondents to assess the quality of pastoral care, a higher proportion of doctors (61 percent) and nurses (56 percent) than of any others gave it an excellent rating.[22] There are occasional misunderstandings between chaplains and doctors. It is likely that many physicians do not quite comprehend the role of the chaplaincy in health care, or do not feel that there is anything for the chaplain to do except when the patient is ready to die.[23] One author politely excuses the doctors by saying that "many physicians wish to administer to the patient's total needs and thus seldom refer patients to chaplains." [24] This implies that the patient has no special spiritual need among the "total needs" cared for by the doctor.

One experienced supervisor of pastoral-care personnel believes the problem of clergy-physician relations is the result of a failure on the part of the chaplains. "Before they can lay claim to professional status," he says, "pastoral care personnel must be able to define their role in terms of the content, the manner, and the purpose of their ministry." Preliminary to this definition, however, is the need for theological reflection about three factors: revelation, the secular, and ambiguity. These three are a "minimum for religious dialogue of any consequence to occur between pastoral personnel and those to whom they are ministering." [25] It appears then that physicians do not understand the chaplain's role, and that frequently the chaplains cannot explain it to them because they themselves are often not sure what they are doing.

One of the frequent irritations expressed about physicians' behavior is that they pass on the unpleasant tasks to the chaplain, for example, to inform the patient that he is terminally ill, or to deal with the family of the patient who has died. These are instances of the "failure" of the medical profession about which the doctor is sometimes embarrassed—as though he were expected to be the arbiter of life and death.[26] Nurses also often note that the doctors "can't take it. They walk away and let us handle the patient in pain, and especially the ones who are dying." The negative complaints about physicians are balanced by positive statements made about nurses in the hospital setting. The general opinion seems to be that the nurses are the "key people" in the care of sick patients. The doctors cannot do without them, and neither can the chaplains. "They are my prime people," said one chaplain. "They are with the patient for long periods of time and they know the patient's needs, spiritual as well as physical. They are my most valuable source of reliable information, and they seem to have genuine personal concern for the sick."

Notes

1 See Joseph H. Fichter, "Pastoral Ministry to the Sick, Suffering, and Dying," *Pastoral Life* 27, no. 5 (May 1978): 2–8; also "Pastoral Care in Catholic Hospitals," *Homiletic and Pastoral Review* 80, no. 7 (April 1980): 32, 50–56.

2 Robert Wheelock and William Walker, "State of the Chaplaincy in Catholic Health Facilities," *Hospital Progress* 53 (September 1972): 38, 40, 42. Earlier emphasis was almost exclusively on medicoethical problems, e.g., Michael Bourke, "A Surgical Code," *Hospital Progress* 1 (May 1920): 36; and Gerald Kelly, "The Moral Code of Catholic Hospitals," *Review for Religious* (July 1953): 205–8.

3 Certification of pastoral associates was not established until

1974, after which growth has been almost spectacular. See Catherine Elliott, *A History of the National Association of Catholic Chaplains* (Washington: NACC, 1975). See the more recent report by Gerald Fath and William Walker, "The 1979 CHA Survey of Pastoral Care Programs," *Hospital Progress* 60 (October 1979): 60–62.

4 Ralph Carr and Walter Smith, "The Catholic Chaplain and Health Care," in *Pastoral Care of the Sick*, ed. the National Association of Catholic Chaplains (Washington: USCC Publication Office, 1974), pp. 39–44.

5 Gerald Kelly, quoted in Robert Shanahan, *The History of the Catholic Hospital Association* (St. Louis: Catholic Hospital Association, 1965) p. 214. See also his brief mention of chaplains, pp. 219–21.

6 Ward A. Knights, "Clinical Preparation for Pastoral Care and Counselling," in *Pastoral Care in Health Facilities* (St. Louis: Catholic Hospital Association, 1977), pp. 4–8.

7 The "founding father" was the Reverend Anton Boisen, *Out of the Depths* (New York: Harper and Brothers, 1960), chap. 5, "An Adventure in Theological Education," pp. 143–97.

8 See the account of St. Mary's Hospital, Rochester, Minnesota, by Cashel Weiler, "Developing a Department of Pastoral Care," *Hospital Progress* 54 (Demember 1973): 42–44. See a more recent account by Anne Corrigan, "Three-year Growth of a Pastoral Care Department," *Hospital Progress* 60 (February 1979): 27–28.

9 Don S. Browning, *The Moral Context of Pastoral Care* (Philadelphia: Westminster, 1976), p. 113.

10 Paul W. Pruyser, *The Minister as Diagnostician* (Philadelphia: Westminster, 1976), p. 54.

11 Spilka's research was described by Cliff Yudell, "Are Clergy Afraid to Die Too?" *U.S. Catholic* (November 1978): 33–39. The research study by B. Spilka, J. Spangler, and M. Rea, "Religion and Death: The Clerical Perspective," was reported at the 1977 Convention of the Society for the Scientific Study of Religion at Chicago, October 30, 1977. A revised version of this paper appears in *Theology Today* 38, no. 1 (April 1981).

12 Robert D. Wheelock, *Health Care Ministries* (St. Louis: Catholic Hospital Association, 1975), p. 54.

13 David M. McPhee, "Women Religious in Pastoral Care," *Hospital Progress* 54 (June 1973): 72–74, 82.

14 See Robert D. Wheelock, *Health Care Ministries* (St. Louis: Catholic Hospital Association, 1975), chap. 9, "Sister-Visitor-Religious Volunteer Program," pp. 58–61. See the report by

118 / Religion and Pain

Rosemary Ellmer, "Lay Volunteers Enlarge Pastoral Care Department's Scope," *Hospital Progress* 61 (May 1980): 78, 80.

15 See Wheelock, *Health Care*, chap. 6, "The Chaplain," pp. 45–50, and chap. 8, "Pastoral Associate," pp. 54–57. In the early years, the chaplains, unlike administrators, physicians, and nurses, were hardly noticed by the Catholic Hospital Association and they remained strictly under "the bishops of the various dioceses in which the hospitals are located." See Robert Shanahan, *The History of the Catholic Hospital Association* (St. Louis: Catholic Hospital Association, 1965), p. 95 and passim.

16 McPhee, "Women Religious," p. 72.

17 Donald L. Worthy, "Hospital Best Setting for Chaplaincy Training," *Hospital Progress* 57 (February 1976): 65–69.

18 Raymond K. Smith, "Training and Certification for Pastoral Care: Is It A Success?" *Hospital Progress* 58 (January 1977): 74–79.

19 Ivan Illich, *Medical Nemesis: The Expropriation of Health* (New York: Bantam Books, 1977), p. 110. See also the special issue of *Daedalus* 106 (Winter 1977), "Doing Better and Feeling Worse: Health in the United States."

20 Harmon L. Smith, "The Minister as Consultant to the Medical Team," *Journal of Religion and Health* 14, no. 1 (January 1975): 7–13.

21 Arnold A. Hutschnecker, *The Will To Live* (New York: Cornerstone Library, 1974), p. 174. See also personal reminiscences of Protestant theologian Donald W. Shriver, in *Medicine and Religion: Strategies for Care*, ed. Donald W. Shriver (Pittsburgh: University of Pittsburgh Press, 1980), pp. 166–68.

22 Raymond Carey, *Hospital Chaplains: Who Needs Them?* (St. Louis: Catholic Hospital Association, 1972), p. 86, concludes that "nurses and doctors clearly put very high value on the services of the chaplain, in fact, higher than the patients do."

23 This reflects the modern notion that often equates health care solely with medical care. Kevin O'Rourke insists that church-related hospitals must integrate pastoral care and medical care. See his article, "Developing a Strong Catholic Identity," *Hospital Progress* 57 (July 1976): 88–90.

24 Cashel Weiler, "Developing a Department of Pastoral Care," *Hospital Progress* 54 (December 1973): 44.

25 Raymond K. Smith, "Theological Reflection on Pastoral Encounter," *Hospital Progress* 57 (March 1976): 78–81.

26 See J. Howard and Anselm Strauss, eds., *Humanizing Health Care* (New York: Wiley, 1975).

Chapter 9

Challenge to Faith

A compelling purpose of organized religion is to bring the "good news" of salvation to all people in the world. All churches engage in evangelization—of their own members as well as of outsiders. At the same time, they want to make a better society, a life of love and justice in which all can participate. Taking care of people in need and in pain is one of the ways to do this. What this means in simple terms is the attempt to build a relationship between God and human beings. All of the so-called apostolates of the organized church—education, health care, missions, retreats, social work—are pointed in this direction. Prayer and worship are a communication with God, but the purpose of apostolic activities is to "fulfill the mission of the pilgrim church to communicate Christ's message through a community of service." [1]

It must be understood, then, that the organized religious response to human pain and suffering is a means of bringing God to people and people to God. Medical care, nursing service, comforting the afflicted—none of these can be an end in itself. Jerome Wilkerson has severely criticized the lack of balance in the health-care apostolate: extraordinary skill is used to preserve and prolong physical life, as though this were more important than to enhance the spiritual element for eternal life. Another author has insisted that church-related hospitals deliver health care primarily as a means to express Christian values. The purpose of the provision of health care is the direct spiritual benefit of the patient.[2] We are told indeed that "Christ, the great physician and healer, cured the whole person—body, mind and spirit. He gave the example that healing and teaching are inseparable." [3] To evangelize is to teach. To ease the burden of pain and sickness is to bring the message of God's love to the suffering patient.

Spiritual Motivation

In attempting to sort out ends and means, we recognize that motivation is multiple and complex. Hospital chaplains of all faiths attest their religious reasons for ministering to the sick. And as we have noted, it is a historical fact that groups of religious women organized themselves precisely to take care of suffering and needy people entirely for spiritual reasons. The respondents to this survey of hospital personnel insist that a spiritual perspective is an essential characteristic of the health-care professional. They agree also that "the holistic approach in modern health care has to include spiritual ministration to patients." In the real world of daily contact between the patient and the medical professional, this spiritual motivation often seems to be in the background—if it is there at all.

In the hospital, the single-minded aim is "let's help these sick people get well, or if they're not getting well, let's ease their pain and give them what comfort we can." Patients have become accustomed to demand relief from pain, to expect that the medical doctor can diagnose what is wrong with them, prescribe proper medication, perform the necessary operation, and otherwise put them "back in shape again." Today people know much more than ever before about preventive medicine and about the steps that can be taken to rehabilitate sick patients. It is a fact also, as some nonbelievers are very quick to point out, that these improvements were introduced by secular medical science, and not by hospital chaplains praying to God on their knees. Research and experimentation in medical laboratories have produced enormous and beneficial results. Progress is still being made through further explorations in hitherto incurable diseases. It is no wonder, then, that the physician has replaced the clergyman, the clinic has replaced the chapel, and the registered nurse has replaced the ordained deaconess. As the Presbyterian chaplain Dennis Saylor writes: "Modern medicine and medical education, in concentrating almost exclusively on scientific concerns, has constructed its own credo: Trust the physician and his medicine." [4]

When interviewing nurses and physicians about their professional training to deal with sick people, we asked them whether they had ever had any lectures, or an academic course, on the spiritual dimensions of health care. Most of the physicians seemed unsure just what the question meant, although they recalled having had some discussion about the ethics of medicine. This is reflected in a statement by a young man just graduating from the Tulane University School of Medicine: "Medical schools seem to want to create robots. That is to say, they ignore personality, emotion, the human spirit, call it what you will. We learn so much about the cistal tubule, and the action of penicillin, and the sounds a sick heart makes, that we never have to pay close attention to what is not mechanical, in patients or in ourselves." [5]

What does spiritual motivation, religious consolation, or sacramental grace mean to a medical doctor whose education has been purely secular and behaviorist? What need does medicine have of spiritual ministry when it is medicine that "gets the results"? Raymond Smith quotes the physician who told the students in a clinical pastoral program: "I examine a patient, and almost always arrive at a diagnosis. I outline a treatment program that includes my part and theirs in it, and I prognosticate a desired result. When *you* are ready to tell me in parallel terms what *you* do in pastoral care, I will accept and welcome you as colleagues in total patient care." [6] This apparently reasonable comparison rests on the not so reasonable assumption that religious ministry can be modeled on medical practice. It also underlines the general problem of the secularist physician's inability to understand humanistic and religious behavior. [7]

The average medical professional does not often allow

himself to be distracted beyond the area of his special competence. The exclusive concentration through years of study on the biological and physiological aspects of the human being has accounted for a certain degree of success in diagnostic capacities, the alleviation of immediate pain and the conquering of disease. On the other hand, more than one veteran doctor has remarked that the success of medical science has been vastly overstated. Franz Ingelfinger writes that "although individual physicians may be well aware of the limitations of medicine and emphasize them, organized medicine on the whole encouraged a belief in the doctor's omniscience rather than his ignorance." [8] The American Medical Association maintains one of the more successful lobbies in the nation's capital and is largely responsible for this pervasive aura of medical omniscience. [9] Of course, not all physicians think of themselves as omniscient, nor are they all so confident of the clear-cut stages from diagnosis to cure. One of them candidly told us: "The youngest and the oldest doctors are impossible to deal with. Before thirty-five they are insecure, uncertain, and threatened by everybody. After fifty-five they feel the progress of science has passed them by and the younger physicians are coming up to take over." Those in the middle-age bracket are confident, affable, and easy to deal with and are among those physicians who "are wont to say that the good doctor does not heal by anything that he does or medicine that he prescribes, but rather tries to establish conditions in which the healing forces of nature can do their work." [10]

The curriculum of medical schools does not include study of the spiritual dimensions of health care, and allows only occasional lectures on medical ethics, at which attendance is not obligatory. The chaplain of a medical school told us that many doctors have real religious faith, "but they have been trained not to show it. They are healers, and should be spiritual healers too. They should know that the touch of their hand is not just a technological touch, but a spiritual touch too. I believe that the training they go through, and the very physicalism of medicine has a tendency to make them materialists, so that God is out of their categories." Although American culture is properly termed "secular," still and all most American adults have had some early contact with an organized religious tradition. Chances are that if they went to Sunday school, their formal religious education ended when they entered high school, though they continued to expand their knowledge in other academic fields, particularly the sciences. Alice O'Shaughnessy remarks that "this is not unique to the medical profession, but the prospect of a competent physician making life-and-death decisions from the religious stance of a fourteen-year-old is disconcerting." [11] The well-trained physician may admit ignorance on an occasional difficult medical case, but in most instances he is probably not educated well enough to recognize his even more flagrant ignorance of religion and spirituality.

We are forced to the conclusion that the great majority of physicians and surgeons—even in church-related hospitals—simply have little or no confidence in the spiritual dimension of sick care. Almost universally they feel that it is "not their business" and they are often embarrassed even to talk about it. Many medical professionals, however, now have a growing concern about the emotional and psychological aspects of pain, and a realization that the healing process goes beyond the anatomical, biological, and physiological. This helps them with problems of psychology, which, however, are still explicable and treatable at the "natural" level of medical care. On the other hand, with relatively few exceptions, medical doctors do not comprehend that spirituality, God, faith, religion—in short the "supernatural"—has any relevance to their primary task of dealing with people in pain.

Women and Spiritual Therapy

Most of what we have said above about medical professionals emerges from research about male physicians and surgeons. Only 7 percent of the medical doctors responding to this hospital survey were women, which is remarkably similar to the small proportion of American women in medicine. We do not know whether this is a representative proportion of women doctors in church-related hospitals, or in hospitals generally. The number of female students in medical school is gradually increasing throughout the country, but they are still a relatively small minority. In all other areas of the health-care profession, the great majority of practitioners are women. Among the 692 respondents to the questionnaire of this study, almost two-thirds (63.7 percent) were females. When we search for the manifestation of spiritual motivation and for the introduction to the religious dimensions of health care, we find that well over half (59 percent) of these female respondents were religious Sisters. Our assumption is that the laywomen do not yet enjoy the depth of spiritual and theological training out of which the religious women operate. We are constrained, then, to comment on the occupational roles—nursing and social work—of both categories of women.

When we query people in these occupations about the faith dimension of health care, do they differ significantly from medical doctors? In discussing the spiritual element of sick care, Mary Kocur remarks: "Nurses have given lip service to 'spiritual care of the patient' for years. There is a chapter in every fundamental nursing text devoted to it. Nurses begin their conventions with a prayer by a chaplain, priest, or minister. Sometimes they pray with and for their patients." [12] She then equates spiritual care with psychic ability and thought control. Nurses of the future may have the responsibility "to teach their patients to meditate and cure themselves of such ailments as hypertension, migraine headaches, and stomach ulcers. Biofeedback is proving such conditions can be cured by learning and applying thought control." There is no indication, however, that student nurses are trained at this sophisticated level, except in some instances when they do graduate study leading to the master's degree.

The nurses we interviewed for this study said generally that they had had some lectures in nursing school concerning medical ethics in relation to patient care. Those who were trained in Catholic schools of nursing also had academic courses in religion, theology, and Scriptures. Living at the nurses' residence, they had frequent contact with religious Sisters and the opportunity for spiritual practices of Mass, communion, prayers, meditation, and retreats. In the contemporary Catholic school of nursing—since the Second Vatican Council—these practices are no longer part of the daily order that the student nurses are expected to follow, but such religious opportunities are available and are announced on the common bulletin board. The Sister director of a Catholic nursing school told us: "Student nurses come here as graduates from high school. We do not have a formal academic course in spirituality, but in the first few weeks as freshmen they are introduced to the fundamentals of nursing. This includes four hours of lectures about the spiritual foundations of nursing. Probably other nursing schools do the same thing. We don't have any particularly Catholic textbook for nursing.[13] Perhaps our philosophy emphasizes more than other schools the spiritual care of the patient as truly deserving of respect and dignity." Later in the conversation she added, "I think also that a Catholic hospital should make a difference, simply because of our faith dimension."

When nurses are asked directly how they bring the comforts of religion to their patients, they often have difficulty articulating their answers. "I am not one to express verbally my religious beliefs. It's more how I express myself nursingwise. It's my sense of care for patients who are suffering. I think that comes across as a form of spirituality." This reply is typical of the remarks made by the Catholic nurses we interviewed, but we always followed up with the question whether religious faith is essential to this kind of health care. "Couldn't this be done by a good sympathetic, non-religious nurse who never goes to church, doesn't even believe in God, but is very compassionate and gives tender, loving care to the patients?" This is, of course, the crucial question that must be answered by all religious believers who say that they are trying to bring God to people in pain. How do they differ from a secular humanist doctor, nurse, or social worker? "The most important thing we do is to give them the support of faith, that suffering must come to an end, and that there is another life beyond this one." This central concept is the spiritual basis on which all the religious believers among the nurses operate, from those who hardly ever mention God and religion, to those who have a zealous missionary and evangelical approach to their patients. While the Nurses Christian Fellowship has a Protestant origin, it is open to ecumenical membership.[14]

There are some males among the social workers who responded to this study, but the majority (73 percent) of them are women. Except for the physicians, the social workers are the least likely among the hospital personnel to say that they pray with and for the sick patients.[15] Their contact with the sick is much less personal than is the case with nurses, and in the larger hospitals they have a great deal of paperwork to do. A sympathetic nursing supervisor commented: "They are so busy filling out the Medicaid and Medicare forms, and explaining why this or that didn't come in yet. That's practically all they do. They're like file clerks. I'm not demeaning their profession, but from a practical point of view they spend so much time making arrangements for monies to be paid to patients." In the smaller hospitals and in places where they have closer contact with the sick, they tend to act as psychological counselors, and in this regard they sometimes think they perform the same role as the pastoral-care personnel.[16] To the extent that they are "secular humanitarians," as Nathan Cohen once characterized American social workers,[17] they are not likely to exercise much spiritual influence on the sick patients. The psychological and spiritual aspects of their patient relations are considered so important that the Catholic Health Association prefers that medical social workers take their graduate studies and professional training at church-related universities.

There is no question, however, that the nurses and social

workers of this study have a greater awareness and concern for the spiritual welfare of their patients than is the case with the medical doctors. These women have lengthier and more frequent contact with the sick and deal with them in a more personal manner than either the physicians or the clergy chaplains. Nurses are particularly able to provide spiritual consolation to the sick.[18] They have been traditionally viewed as "angels of mercy," and many of them strive to continue this role in spite of the mechanization and depersonalization of the modern hospital.

Chaplains and the Faith

At some ideal level, all of the personnel in a church-related hospital are seen as a community of health service which includes the healing service of faith. Everyone is supposed in some way or another to bring the comforts of religion to people in pain. We have questioned to what extent this is accomplished and we have seen that the spiritual dimension of health care tends to take second place to the specific medical or physical roles. The only person who has a direct mandate to bring God to the patient and to construct, or reinforce, the divine-human relationship is the chaplain. Traditionally in the larger hospitals the chaplain had an office, which he hardly ever used, and out of which he made daily rounds of visiting patients. He was always within reach for an emergency call. The modern chaplain is a member of the pastoral-care department, which normally includes female pastoral associates.[19] The pastoral role is now officially labeled "professional" because the chaplain has gone through a training period and has been accredited either by the Protestant Association of Clinical Pastoral Education or by the Office of Chaplain Services of the United States Catholic Conference. Thus, the individual is qualified by tested professional competence, and not by ordination, or by vows of religion, or by appointment of an ecclesiastical official.

The decision to switch from the old-style chaplaincy to the new department of pastoral care must be made by the hospital administration. One observer has gone so far as to say that pastoral care should be looked upon "as a management service similar to purchasing, data processing, and fiscal services, now made available to hospitals." It seems odd to make this kind of comparison, and to put pastoral care on the same level as these mundane services, especially in a church-related hospital, but the challenge is made that until this is done, "the development of pastoral care departments will continue to be haphazard." [20]

Seminaries and schools of theology now assign their students, both male and female, to a period of "field work" in hospitals and clinics. For most of them, this is simply part of the professional preparation for future ministry, which may involve little more than an occasional visit to sick parishioners. At best, it is a useful experience that gives them a perspective on the specialized hospital ministry. Most of the chaplains who answered our questionnaire, however, and all of those we interviewed, had had no field work of this kind when they were in divinity school. But of most importance to the central concern of this study is the fact that the modern members of the departments of pastoral care have had thorough theological training. They possess the content of the spiritual role they now perform. Their ministry is to communicate God's message of love and salvation to sick people. Since the holistic approach includes, by definition, the spiritual dimension of health care, they are cooperating in the team ministry for the bodily, psychological, and spiritual welfare of the sick patients.

The chaplains who answered this survey think of themselves as members of a team involved in the entire process of caring for the patient. They repudiate the notion that "religion is a kind of last resort when medical science is unable to relieve pain." Like Paul Pruyser, they repudiate also the generalization that "where the doctor leaves off or has to admit his failure, the priest's or minister's work begins." [21] Religion is supposed to be present throughout the whole period of sickness, not only in the terminal phase when some kind of magic intervention is sought. The healing process reaches beyond the bodily dimension but should not be separated from it. Both the pastoral and the medical personnel are integral to the team and should be in support of each other. "If the spiritual values conveyed to patients by the pastoral care department are not reinforced by the medical personnel's attitudes and concerns, the hospital as a whole becomes a dichotomy, with spiritual values and human professionalism in sharp contrast."[22]

No matter how sympathetic we may be with the stated ideals of church-related hospitals and with the zealous dedication of chaplains and pastoral associates, we must, nevertheless, conclude that at the present time spiritual values are secondary to the advanced technical status of hospitals. We are told that the "fundamental responsibility" is fourfold: to promote health, to prevent illness, to restore health, and to alleviate suffering. The challenge to religious faith is that spiritual motivation be at the basis of professional responsibility, and that the spiritual dimension of health care be taken seriously in the ministry to the sick. Up to now, and in most hospitals, it has been our observation that pastoral assistants, ministers, and clergy, if they are admitted to membership on the "team," are generally still kept at the edge of the group, but this state of affairs is rapidly changing.

Notes

1 See William Kenney and Charles Ceronsky, "Developing Christian Values in a Catholic Health Facility," *Hospital Progress* 55 (October 1974): 32, 36–37.

2 Jerome F. Wilkerson, "Aggiornamento: Dedication of Religious in Maintaining Catholic Hospitals," *Hospital Progress* 46 (July 1965): 75–76. See also Sr. Mary Brigh, "Purpose and Need of Church-sponsored Health Facilities," *Hospital Progress* 49 (September 1968): 59–60.

3 C. M. Frank, *Foundations of Nursing* (Philadelphia: Saunders, 1959), chap. 3, "The Influence of Christianity on the Healing

Arts," pp. 31–40. See also Bernard Martin, *The Healing Ministry of the Church* (Richmond: John Knox Press, 1961).

4 Dennis Saylor, *And You Visited Me* (Medford: Morse Press, 1979), p. 197. For a broader perspective, see Stanley Reiser, *Medicine and the Reign of Technology* (New York: Cambridge University Press, 1978).

5 Ned Hallowell, "The Message from the Dais," Commencement, 1978, *The Tulanian* (Summer 1978): 6. See also John Bryant, "Obstacles to Change in Medical Education," *World Medical Journal* 20 (1973): 33–36.

6 Raymond K. Smith, "Theological Reflection on Pastoral Encounter," *Hospital Progress* 57 (March 1976): 78–81.

7 For an effort to remedy this kind of misapprehension, see William Rogers and David Barnard, eds., *Nourishing the Humanistic in Medicine: Interaction with the Social Sciences* (Pittsburgh: University of Pittsburgh Press, 1978). For a wider concern, see Daniel Callahan, "Health and Society: Some Ethical Imperatives," *Daedalus*, 106 (Winter 1977): 23–33.

8 Franz J. Ingelfinger, "Medicine: Meritorious or Meretricious," *Science* 200 (26 May 1978): 942–46. See also the cynical reflections of Robert Mendelsohn, *Confessions of a Medical Heretic* (New York: Warner, 1980).

9 One of the better-known authors who discusses this topic is Richard Harris, *A Sacred Trust* (Baltimore: Penguin, 1969). Again, the most vitriolic attack is that of Ivan Illich, *Medical Nemesis: The Expropriation of Health* (New York: Pantheon, 1976).

10 Harry C. Meserve, "Religion's Contribution to Health," *Journal of Religion and Health* 13, no. 1 (January 1974): 3–5.

11 Alice O'Shaughnessy, "The Role of Religion in Patient Care," in *Medicine and Religion: Strategies of Care*, ed. Donald W. Shriver, Jr. (Pittsburgh: University of Pittsburgh Press, 1980), pp. 99–105.

12 Mary D. Kocur, "Health Care in the 1980s," *Hospital Progress* 55 (January 1974): 62, 65–66. In some respects, the work of the nurse "is akin to that of the minister" says Pastor Heije Faber, *Pastoral Care in the Modern Hospital* (Philadelphia: Westminster Press, 1977), p. 101.

13 She named the textbook used in this nursing school: Beverly W. DuGas, *Introduction to Patient Care*, 3rd ed. (Philadelphia: Saunders, 1977).

14 Members of the Nurses Christian Fellowship are deeply

spiritual women who find guidance in the work of Sharon Fish and Judith Shelley, *Spiritual Care: The Nurse's Role* (Downers Grove: Intervarsity Press, 1978)

15 See Carleton Pilsecker, "Help for the Dying," *Social Work* 20 (May 1975): 190–94, who omits any mention of religion in the role of the social worker with the terminally ill patient or his family.

16 See the response of Robert Wheelock to the charge that hospital chaplains are simply duplicating the functions of medical social workers. "Is Pastoral Care Health Care?" *Hospital Progress* 56 (May 1975): 38, 40.

17 Cited by Herbert Stroup, "The Common Predicament of Religion and Social Work," *Social Work* 7 (April 1962): 89–93.

18 Raymond Carey suggests that nurses are "at a disadvantage" because they cannot counsel as well as chaplains and do not know the patient as well as doctors. See his "Living Unitl Death," *Hospital Progress* 55 (February 1974): 82–87.

19 See David M. McPhee, "Women Religious in Pastoral Care," *Hospital Progress* 54 (June 1973): 72–74, 82.

20 John W. Mullally, CHSLP Pastoral Care Model: A Response," *Hospital Progress* 56 (July 1975): 78–80, 82.

21 Paul W. Pruyser, *The Minister as Diagnostician* (Philadelphia: Westminster, 1976), p. 42.

22 Cornelius J. Van Der Poel, "Teamwork Integrates Professionalism and Pastoral Care," *Hospital Progress* 58 (January 1977): 64–67.

Appendix

Questionnaire

An Enquiry about Spiritual Ministry to the Sick

1. As a professional in the field of health care you are daily faced with the problem of pain and suffering and you do all you can to relieve it.

2. Each person in this field has a specific contribution to make for the welfare of the patient. We are asking to what extent there is also a religious, or spiritual, approach to the suffering person.

3. We appreciate the fact that you are a busy person and we have tried to make the responses as convenient as possible. Most of them can be made by a check-off in the appropriate parenthesis ( ).

4. Please take the time to answer these questions as frankly as you can, and return your answers in the enclosed postpaid envelope.

5. In general, how is spiritual ministry to the sick rated in this hospital?
   ( ) High rating   ( ) Medium   ( ) Low

6–9. Do the ministers of religion get full cooperation here from:
   Hospital administration   ( ) Yes   ( ) No
   Nurses and aides   ( ) Yes   ( ) No
   Physicians and surgeons   ( ) Yes   ( ) No
   Social service workers   ( ) Yes   ( ) No

10. Does this hospital have a Department of Pastoral Care?
    ( ) Yes   ( ) No
    If yes, how many full-time members are on it? _____

11. What is your general assessment of pastoral care at this hospital?
    ( ) Excellent   ( ) Pretty good   ( ) Only fair

133

12. Please estimate roughly what proportion of the patients here are:

    (%) Catholics   (%) Protestants   (%) Others

13. What is your own occupation or professional position at this hospital?

    ( ) Chaplain   ( ) Nurse   ( ) Physician
    ( ) Social Worker   ( ) _____

14. Do you consider spiritual ministry to the sick an aspect of *your own work?*

    It is: ( ) Essential   ( ) Occasional   ( ) Peripheral

15–28. Here is a series of statements one sometimes hears from people who are dealing with the sick. Please indicate your own opinion on each by circling one of the letters: (SA) strongly agree; (A) agree; (N) neither agree nor disagree; (D) disagree; (SD) strongly disagree.

15. You can't be a good health professional unless you have a spiritual perspective on life   SA   A   N   D   SD

16. Pain and suffering are God's way of punishing us for our sins   SA   A   N   D   SD

17. The holistic approach in modern health care has to include spiritual ministration to patients   SA   A   N   D   SD

18. In the long run, all healing is attributable to the providence of God   SA   A   N   D   SD

19. Faith in God lessens the fears and anxieties of the suffering person   SA   A   N   D   SD

20. The Bible teaches us that God does not really want us to suffer   SA   A   N   D   SD

21. Advances in medical science will someday allow us to alleviate all physical pain   SA   A   N   D   SD

22. Physicians and nurses should not be expected to talk about God with their patients   SA   A   N   D   SD

23. Prayer is a helpful part of the healing process for people in pain   SA   A   N   D   SD

24. Religious faith provides the ultimate meaning to the mystery of suffering   SA   A   N   D   SD

25. The more religious a person is the more able he or she is to endure suffering   SA A N D SD

26. Religion is a kind of last resort when medical science is unable to relieve pain   SA A N D SD

27. In the hospital setting no one but a clergyman should talk about religion to the patient   SA A N D SD

28. Suffering chronic pain has no meaning unless one believes in God   SA A N D SD

29. Which of the following terms fits your current status:
    - ( ) Diocesan priest
    - ( ) Religious priest
    - ( ) Permanent deacon
    - ( ) Religious Brother
    - ( ) Religious Sister
    - ( ) Lay woman
    - ( ) Lay man

30. What is your highest academic, or professional, degree? _____

31. How long have you been in the health care profession? _____ years

32. How long have you been employed at this hospital? _____ years

33. Have you ever seen a case of "miraculous" remission (that is, one that was unexpected, or unexplained by doctors)?
    ( ) Yes   ( ) No

    If yes, please describe briefly: _____

34. Would you describe yourself as:
    - ( ) Quite religious
    - ( ) Somewhat
    - ( ) Not very
    - ( ) Hardly at all

35. What is your religious (or church) affiliation? _____

36. If you could make the choice over again, would you still choose this same occupation or profession?
    - ( ) Yes, definitely
    - ( ) Probably yes
    - ( ) Probably no
    - ( ) Definitely no

37–45. This series of statements tends to be very personal. Please indicate your agreement or disagreement.

37. I am not competent to talk religion with patients   SA A N D SD

38. My approach to health care is technical   SA   A   N   D   SD

39. I pray for God's guidance in my work   SA   A   N   D   SD

40. Experience with sick people brings me close to God   SA   A   N   D   SD

41. I regularly pray for my patients   SA   A   N   D   SD

42. The suffering I see every day weakens my faith   SA   A   N   D   SD

43. Sometimes I pray with the sick people   SA   A   N   D   SD

44. I get depressed when a patient dies   SA   A   N   D   SD

45. Physicians here tend to belittle spiritual ministry   SA   A   N   D   SD

46. How many women religious (Sisters) are on the staff here?

    _____

47–52. How many of the Sisters are in each of the following positions:

    ( ) Supervisors   ( ) Bedside nurses   ( ) Pastoral care

53. Is there a Pain Clinic attached to this hospital?

    ( ) No   ( ) Yes, but I am not involved in it
    ( ) Yes, I work in it

54. Please write here the name and address of this hospital:

    _____

    _____

55. If you would like to receive a personal copy of the report of this survey please provide your own name and address:

    _____

    _____

NOTE: You are very kind in taking the trouble to answer this questionnaire. Feel free to add any comments or recommendations on the back of this page. May the Lord bless you and the important work you do for sick people.

Joseph H. Fichter

Index

137